MAJOR INCIDENT MEDICAL MANAGEMENT AND SUPPORT

MAJOR INCIDENT MEDICAL MANAGEMENT AND SUPPORT

The Practical Approach

Advanced Life Support Group

BMJ
Publishing
Group

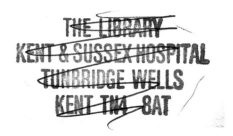
© BMJ Publishing Group 1995

First published 1995

British Library Cataloguing in Publication Data
A catalogue record for this book is available from the British Library

ISBN 0-7279-0928-2

Typeset, printed, and bound in Great Britain by
Latimer Trend & Company Ltd, Plymouth

PREFACE

"It couldn't happen to us" is not an acceptable excuse for being ill prepared to deal with a major incident. A major incident may occur at any time, anywhere.

Guidelines exist for the Health Services' response to a major incident and these cover both the hospital and the scene. Each hospital must have its own major incident plan and this should be exercised regularly. How well do we teach the principles of the major incident response to our medical and nursing staff? How much do we learn from our exercises? Are mistakes being repeated?

It is no longer acceptable to approach the scene of a major incident as an enthusiastic amateur. The transition from working in the emergency department to working at the scene does not simply involve putting on a reflective jacket and a pair of Wellington boots. The medical service must, like the Police, Fire, and Ambulance Services, be skilled in command and communications, and have experience of the pre-hospital environment. This is in addition to coping with the enormous strain that mass casualties will place on the medical resources. To do this requires knowledge and training.

This manual, although a stand alone text, has been prepared to accompany a course structured to teach the principles of management and support at a major incident to Health Service staff. The course will prepare both the incident officers and other members of the scene medical response for their duties in the event of a major incident.

TJ Hodgetts
K Mackway-Jones
(*Editors*)
Manchester

August 1995

ACKNOWLEDGMENTS

The authors wish to thank Ian Dearden, Karen Gwinnutt, and Susan Wieteska for their assistance with preparing the text.

We are indebted yet again to Mary Harrison and Helen Carruthers for their excellent line diagrams which accompany the text.

We must also thank candidates involved in the pilot courses for their constructive comments, in particular Mr Peter Bedford who spent considerable time helping us by scanning the text thoroughly.

Note

Throughout most of this text the male gender is used, where either male or female applies. In addition it has not always been possible to avoid use of terms, such as ambulanceman, manpower, man made, which could be construed as sexist. We ask the reader not to take offence—this has been done to avoid ambiguity or cumbersome sentence construction.

CONTENTS

CONTENTS

WORKING GROUP

Matthew Cooke, Emergency Medicine, Birmingham

Robert Cocks, Emergency Medicine, London

Timothy Hodgetts, Emergency Medicine, RAMC

Colville Laird, Immediate Care, Auchterarder, Scotland

Kevin Mackway-Jones, Emergency Medicine, Manchester

John Scott, Immediate Care, Cambridge

EDITORS

Timothy J Hodgetts, MRCP, DipIMC, RCSEd, Emergency Medicine, Royal Army Medical Corps

Kevin Mackway-Jones, MRCP, FRCS, FFAEM, Emergency Medicine, Manchester

CONTRIBUTORS

Christopher Cahill, Emergency Medicine, Royal Navy

Matthew Cooke, Emergency Medicine, Birmingham

Patrick Corocoran, Fire and Rescue Service, Manchester

Simon Davies, Emergency Nursing, Stoke on Trent

Peter Driscoll, Emergency Medicine, Manchester

Kenneth Dunn, Burns Surgery, Manchester

Stephen Hawes, Emergency Medicine, Manchester

Timothy Hodgetts, Emergency Medicine, Royal Army Medical Corps

Philip Jones, Ambulance Service, Manchester

Colville Laird, Immediate Care, Auchterarder

Kevin Mackway-Jones, Emergency Medicine, Manchester

Geoffrey Pike, Fire and Rescue Service, Manchester

Stephen Southworth, Emergency Medicine, Manchester

David Ward, Emergency Planning, North West Region

PART

I

INTRODUCTION

Major incidents: a history and overview

This chapter provides a historical perspective of major incidents and will answer the following questions:

- What is a major incident?
- What are the objectives for major incident medical management and support?
- How can we prepare ourselves for a major incident?
- What are our priorities at the scene of a major incident?

DEFINING A MAJOR INCIDENT

The Health Service definition of a major incident cannot be stated simply in terms of the total number of live or dead casualties. It must also reflect the ability of the service to cope with whatever number of *live* casualties there are, using the resources available in normal daily working practice (Box 1.1). Twenty casualties distributed evenly among four hospitals within a metropolitan area may produce only a ripple in the delivery of emergency health care. If all 20 casualties were taken to an isolated rural hospital its practice might be disrupted for many days or weeks.

Box 1.1. Health service definition of a major incident

A health service major incident is said to exist when:

- Any occurrence presents a serious threat to the health of the community
- The health service is disrupted
- There are, or are likely to be, so many casualties that special arrangements are necessary to deal with them

---

On 2 September 1666 a fire started in a baker's shop on Pudding Lane; it lasted four days and left 80% of London's buildings in ruins. A disaster on such a scale is hard to imagine and would certainly overwhelm the resources of the modern Fire Service. Miraculously only a handful of people died in this, the Great Fire of London.

On 22 December 1988 a terrorist device aboard Pan Am flight 103 exploded as the aircraft flew over the borders of England and Scotland. All 259 passengers and crew on board died, together with 11 inhabitants of Lockerbie. Few people were injured.

If the definition shown in Box 1.1 is applied to either the Great Fire of London or the Lockerbie air crash then neither can be considered to have been a major incident in Health Service terms. Both these incidents were, undoubtedly, major incidents for other emergency services, and continued to strain the resources of the local authorities for many months after the event.

It is important to note that the precise nature of an incident may take some time to become clear, and that activation of Health Service procedures will occur when the definition is not fulfilled. This over-reaction is unavoidable.

> **A major incident for one emergency service may not apply to all emergency services**

The Police and Fire Service define a major incident as shown in Box 1.2.

Box 1.2. Police and Fire Service definitions of a major incident

A major incident is said to exist when special arrangements are necessary for:

- The initial treatment, rescue, and transport of large numbers of casualties
- The direct or indirect involvement of large numbers of people
- The handling of a large number of enquiries from both the public and the media (usually to the Police)
- The need for the large scale combined resources of the three emergency services
- The mobilisation and organisation of the emergency services and supporting organisations, for example, the local authority, to cater for the threat of death, serious injury, or homelessness to a large number of people

---

Major incident or major disaster?

These two terms are often used loosely and interchangeably. It is recommended, however, that the term "disaster" be reserved for events that produce a wider disturbance in the community, other than the need for special arrangements by the emergency services—for example, an earthquake or flood.

Classification of major incidents

It is convenient to classify major incidents in two ways:

1 Compensated or uncompensated
2 Simple or compound.

A *compensated* incident is one in which the casualties can be dealt with by mobilising additional resources, that is, the "load is less than the capacity." An example is the Clapham rail disaster in 1988, where the 115 injured were treated by paramedics, immediate care doctors, and hospital Mobile Medical Teams at the scene, and transported to a number of hospitals for definitive treatment. An *uncompensated* incident occurs when the additional medical resources mobilised by instituting major incident plans are still inadequate to cope with the number of casualties, that is, the "load exceeds the capacity"—examples occur in *natural* disasters such as an earthquake (Table 1.1), or flood, in which case these disasters often are also "compound" (see below); however, *man made* incidents may occasionally be of such a magnitude that they exceed the capacity of the health resources (as happened in Bhopal, India, on 3 December 1984 when the valve on a tank of methyl isocyanate burst, releasing a toxic cloud which killed an estimated 3000–10 000 and left 500 000 disfigured or disabled).

4

Table 1.1. Earthquakes, ancient and modern

Date	Place	Estimated casualties
AD 526	Antioch, Syria	250 000*
18 April 1906	San Francisco	1000 injured
1 September 1923	Tokyo	150 000*
28 July 1976	T'angshan, China	655 000*
19 September 1985	Mexico City	40 000*
7 December 1988	Armenia	55 000*

* Dead.

In an uncompensated incident, the load of live casualties is greater than the capacity of the system

---

In a *simple* incident the infrastructure remains intact—that is, the roads, the hospitals, and the lines of communication. Most incidents that occur in the Western World fall into this category. When this infrastructure is damaged, by a natural disaster or by war, then the incident is said to be *compound*. Even the best made incident plans will be ineffective if the hospitals are part of the disaster.

In a compound disaster the infrastructure is destroyed

Types of major incident

As already implied, major incidents may also be categorised as natural or man made.

Natural—A *natural* disaster is the result of earthquake, flood, tsunami (seismic tidal wave), volcano, drought, famine, or pestilence (Tables 1.1 and 1.2). To some extent the natural disaster will be self propagating—following a flood or earthquake, those left homeless and starving will be vulnerable to the diseases associated with squalor. In September 1887 the Yellow River in China (nicknamed "China's Sorrow"—it has caused more deaths than any other natural feature in the world) burst its banks flooding 11 cities and hundreds of villages in the Henan Province; 900 000 died following the flood, and almost one million more died from the subsequent famine and disease.

Table 1.2. Natural disasters

Date	Place	Estimated dead
24 August 79	Pompeii and Herculaneum (eruption of Vesuvius)	20 000
28 December 1908	Straits of Messina (tsunami destroying Messina and Reggio)	160 000
4 April 1927	Mississippi river (flood)	300
12 November 1970	Bangladesh (cyclone)	200 000
18 September 1974	Honduras (Hurricane Fifi)	3 000
6 June 1980	Dallas, Texas (heat wave)	1 200
11 November 1985	Columbia (Nevada del Reuiz volcano)	25 000

Man made—The diversity of man made incidents is very broad, but certain patterns are clear. The ingredients are present for a major incident when large numbers of people gather together to work, to travel, or for leisure. In some circumstances the incident will be a result of a deliberate terrorist activity. We will consider examples of man made incidents under the headings of industrial, transport, sporting, and terrorist (Tables 1.3–1.6).

Industrial incidents—The mining industry has provided a number of industrial major incidents (Table 1.3).

Table 1.3. Industrial incidents

Date	Place	Estimated casualties
14 October 1913	Senghenydd coal mine, Wales (explosion)	439*
21 October 1966	Aberfan, Wales (slag heap land slip)	147*
2 May 1972	Sunshine silver mine, Idaho (fire)	91*
6 July 1988	Piper Alpha rig, North Sea (explosion)	164*
		25 + injured

* Dead.

Perhaps the most frightening industrial incident to date (a true *disaster*) has been the explosion of a nuclear reactor at Chernobyl in Russia on 5 April 1986, which left much of Europe contaminated with radioactive material. Around 40 000 inhabitants of Chernobyl were exposed to phenomenal levels of radiation for six days. The official estimates of 31 dead, 1000 injured, and 6000 losing their lives to cancer in the subsequent 70 years are likely to be gross underestimates.

To some extent the consequences of an industrial incident can be predicted. Strict guidelines exist for emergency planning at fixed chemical and nuclear installations, and for the management of contaminated casualties.

Transport incidents—Virtually all forms of transport boast an impressive list of associated major incidents (Table 1.4). The worst ever road traffic accident occurred in the Salang tunnel in Afghanistan in 1982 when a petrol tanker exploded. Such was the degree of destruction that only an estimate could be made of the number of dead as between 1100 and 2700.

Table 1.4. Transport incidents

Date	Type	Place	Casualties
11 April 1912	Sea	Sinking of *Titanic*	1403*
3 May 1937	Airship	New Jersey (Hindenberg explodes)	36*
8 October 1952	Rail crash	Harrow	112*
28 February 1975	London Underground	Moorgate	43*; 74 injured
November 1982	Road	Salang tunnel fire	2700* (approx.)
22 August 1985	Aircraft fire	Manchester	55*; 80 injured
6 March 1987	Sea	Zeebrugge, *Herald of Free Enterprise* capsizes	137*; 402 injured
9 September 1987	Road	M4 motorway	4*; 74 injured
18 November 1987	London Underground	King's Cross (fire)	31*; 60 injured
12 December 1988	Rail crash	Clapham Junction	34*; 115 injured
22 December 1988	Aircraft bomb	Lockerbie	270*
8 January 1989	Aircraft crash	Kegworth (M1)	47*; 79 injured

* Dead.

Sporting incidents—Any crowd is vulnerable to the effects of crush, but some of the worst tragedies have occurred at football stadia around the world (Table 1.5). The reasons have included: an overfull stadium (Bolton 1946; Hillsborough 1989); a dejected home crowd surging back into the stadium with a last minute goal (Moscow 1982—these figures were not released until 1989); or a crowd escaping a hailstorm (Kathmandu 1988). Recent events in the United Kingdom have prompted reviews of the safety of football stadia and the statutory medical cover for such events, published in the Taylor and Gibson reports respectively.

Table 1.5. Sporting incidents (football)

Date	Place	Casualties
UK		
9 March 1946	Burnden Park, Bolton (crush)	33*; 400 injured
2 January 1971	Ibrox, Glasgow (crush)	66*; 100 injured
11 May 1985	Bradford City Stadium (fire)	55*; 200 injured
15 April 1989	Hillsborough, Sheffield (crush)	95*; 200 injured
International		
24 May 1964	Lima, Peru (crush)	318*; 500 injured
20 October 1982	Moscow (crush)	340*
29 May 1985	Heysel Stadium, Brussels (crush)	41*; 437 injured
March 1988	Kathmandu, Nepal (crush)	100*; 300 injured
13 January 1991	Orkney, South Africa (riot)	40*; 50 injured

* Dead.

Terrorism—It is unfortunate that terrorism is responsible for an increasing number of deaths and injuries, and it is the terrorist bomb that has regularly produced multiple casualties on such a scale. The first Irish terrorist bomb in Britain occurred in 1867 at the Clerkenwell House of Detention in London, when an attempt was made to spring Fenian prisoners (Table 1.6). Some 10 000 people are estimated to have been killed or injured in the last two decades by terrorist bombs.

Table 1.6. Terrorist incidents

Date	Place	Casualties
13 December 1867	London	15*; 40 injured
5 October 1974	Birmingham (*Horse and Groom*)	5*; 62 injured
21 November 1974	Birmingham (*Tavern in the Town*)	11*; 89 injured
8 November 1987	Enniskillin	11*; 60 injured
10 April 1992	City of London	3*; 93 injured
20 March 1993	Warrington	2*; 55 injured

* Dead.

It can be seen that each major incident may produce a disproportionate number of casualties with similar injuries such as burns (Bradford City and King's Cross fires); hypothermia and drowning (*Herald of Free Enterprise*); traumatic asphyxia (football stadia disasters); and blast injury (terrorist bombs). A spectacular example of this is the Ramstein airshow disaster on 28 August 1988, when aerobatic jets collided and plunged into the crowd injuring 530 (predominantly with burns) and killing 34.

HEALTH SERVICE OBJECTIVES

Major Incident Medical Management and Support (MIMMS) provides a structured approach to the major incident scene (major incident medical *management*) and to dealing with multiple casualties (major incident medical *support*). This approach can

7

be adopted by the Health Services Incident Officers and by all other members of the Health Services involved in the response.

The main objectives of the Health Services are to do the following:

- Save life
- Prevent further harm to the injured
- Relieve suffering.

The medical services must work closely with the Ambulance Service to achieve these aims.

PREPARING FOR A MAJOR INCIDENT

There are three elements to medical preparation for a major incident:

1 Planning
2 Equipment
3 Training.

These will be dealt with in detail in subsequent chapters.

Planning

Every hospital that is equipped to receive casualties must have a Major Incident Plan, and this plan should include the provision of a Mobile Medical Team, as well as detailing the individual actions of key hospital personnel. The plan should be reviewed and updated if faults are detected when it is exercised.

Equipment

Both the Incident Officers and all medical and nursing staff at the scene should wear adequate personal protective equipment. The nature of this is dealt with in Chapter 9. The response should include mobilisations of equipment matched to the skills of the responders; this is dealt with in Chapter 10.

In addition, staff must be provided with communications equipment and must be familiar with its use.

Training

There are two aspects to training: education and exercise. It is recommended that only personnel who have received training be expected to perform the roles of Medical Incident Officer, or Ambulance Incident Officer, and that all members of Mobile Medical Teams are adequately trained.

The principles of patient assessment and treatment are those taught on the Advanced Life Support Courses: these skills will be essential to members of the medical team, but must be applied appropriately to the pre-hospital setting.

Paper exercises within the hospital should take place at least every six months to highlight administrative problems. Independent of these the emergency department can perform paper *triage* exercises. On an annual basis the hospital should practise the plan in full; this can be done either as a table top exercise using a model, or as a combined exercise with the emergency services in a simulated disaster (Box 1.3). Individual emergency services, particularly the Fire Service, regularly exercise on a smaller scale, and it is possible to become involved with them so as to maintain the level of training throughout the year, and to give a number of people the opportunity to take the role of the Incident Officer.

Box 1.3. Types of major incident exercise

Paper exercise
Table top exercise
Departmental exercise
Interservice exercise

Training is dealt with in more detail in Appendix C.

The elements of good preparation for a major incident are planning, training, and equipment

---

THE SCENE RESPONSE

When faced with the chaotic scene of a major incident it is important that order is brought about rapidly. This book recommends a structured approach which will enable Incident Officers to initiate and later develop a series of events that will provide the best medical care for the injured. The principles can be applied to the management of both single casualty accidents and major incidents.

The management and support priorities for the emergency health services are listed in Box 1.4.

Box 1.4. Management and support priorities

Command
Safety
Communications
Assessment
Triage
Treatment
Transport

These priorities can usefully be remembered with the mnemonic:

Control Spells Calm And Time To Treat

Thus Incident Officers must take *command* of resources—as dealt with in detail in Chapters 12 and 13.

All health personnel are responsible for their own safety, for the safety of the scene, and for the safety of individual casualties. The Safety Officers will oversee this on behalf of the Incident Officers. The 1–2–3 of safety is shown in Box 1.5.

Box 1.5. 1–2–3 of safety

1 Yourself
2 The scene
3 The casualties

Communications between the Ambulance, Police, and Fire Incident Officers must be established early, and arrangements made for regular liaison. Radios will be available from the Ambulance Emergency Control Vehicle (ECV), and staff there will confirm the call signs of key personnel. The main failing of major incident management is poor communications. Communications are dealt with in Chapters 11 and 20.

The main failing of major incident management is poor communications

A rapid *assessment* of the scene (for significant hazards and to estimate the number and severity of injured) is essential. The information gathered is used to determine the initial medical response needed at the scene and to brief the hospitals (via the ECV) about how many casualties they can expect.

Triage is the sorting of casualties into priorities for treatment. The process is dynamic (priorities may alter after treatment or while waiting for treatment), and it must be repeated at every stage of the evacuation chain to detect these changes. A system for triage is given in Chapter 16. The triage priorities are listed in Table 1.7.

Table 1.7. Triage priorities

Priority	Colour	Label	
IMMEDIATE	Red	P1	T1
URGENT	Yellow	P2	T2
DELAYED	Green	P3	T3
EXPECTANT	Blue (green if no blue label)		T4
DEAD	White/black		

P, priority; T, treatment.

The aim of treatment at a major incident is to "do the most for the most," that is, to identify and treat the salvageable. Actual treatment delivered will reflect the skills of the services as well as the environment. Treatment is dealt with further in Chapter 17, and practical procedures are detailed in Chapters 21, 22, and 23.

Transport to hospital is the responsibility of the Ambulance Incident Officer who will determine which hospital the patient is sent to, and by which route. The aim of evacuation at a major incident is to get

"the **right patient** to the **right place** in the **right time**."

Transport is dealt with in detail in Chapter 18.

Members of the Mobile Medical Team will not be directly involved with *command* or scene *assessment* (other than assessing any hazards in the area where they are working).

THE HOSPITAL RESPONSE

The principal objective of the Medical and Ambulance Incident Officers at the scene is to get the injured to a definitive care facility as soon as possible. This does not simply mean taking all the patients to the nearest hospital because this will overwhelm their resources. A number of pulses of patients should be sent to a number of "receiving" hospitals so as to spread the load. It may be appropriate to evacuate patients from the scene directly to a specialist centre, if, for example, they had an isolated head injury or severe burns.

> **The Mobile Medical Team(s) should not come from the main receiving hospital(s)**

At the hospital the principle of prioritising for treatment (triage) will be continued. Departmental reorganisation will be required to cope with large numbers of seriously injured. Areas will be designated in the Major Incident Plan to receive priority 1, 2, and 3 patients and the staffing levels these areas will require will be specified. Patients will need to be moved or discharged from acute wards. A central control room will coordinate the hospital response. A fuller description of the hospital response is given in Chapter 15.

THE AFTERMATH

The pre-hospital phase will often last only several hours. The additional strain on an individual hospital will be felt for many days or even weeks. The rehabilitation of some patients can take years.

Most of the hospital staff and many of the emergency service personnel will never have experienced such an event, and understandably some will show signs of stress. This may be immediate and occur during the incident, but this is much less common than an insidious syndrome of reliving the events with flashbacks and nightmares, resulting in anxiety, sleeplessness, and poor performance at work. This syndrome is known as the "post-traumatic stress disorder" (PTSD). Psychological aspects of disasters are discussed in Appendix B.

> **Summary**
> - A major incident has occurred when the number, severity, type, or location of live casualties require extraordinary arrangements by the Health Service
> - Major incidents can be simple or compound, compensated or uncompensated, and natural or man made
> - Most major incidents are simple, compensated, and man made
> - MIMMS provides a structured approach to the medical management of the scene of a major incident, and to the medical support of multiple casualties. This can be applied by all members of the health services at the scene

2

Guidance and requirements

After reading this chapter you should be able to answer the following questions:

- What guidance is available for the emergency services and other agencies?
- What specific guidance exists for the NHS response?
- What does the NHS guidance say?

INTRODUCTION

Each of the emergency services has different responsibilities in the event of a major incident involving large numbers of casualties. These are discussed in more detail in later chapters. In broad terms, the Police are concerned with the control of the incident site, the maintenance of law and order, the preservation of evidence, and investigation of the cause. The Fire Service are concerned with rescue and containment of hazards such as fire, chemical, and radioactive contamination. The Ambulance and Medical Services are concerned with the saving and preservation of life both at the scene and subsequently at receiving hospitals. Other agencies such as local authorities, industry, volunteer organisations, and the military may also become involved. It is essential that everyone involved has a single set of aims and objectives. A key piece of guidance is that there should be a combined response to major incident management. The objectives of this combined response have been described as in Box 2.1.

Box 2.1. Objectives of the combined response

Save life
Prevent escalation of the incident
Relieve suffering
Protect the environment
Protect property
Rapidly restore normality
Facilitate enquiries

Immediate care of victims

Immediate care and treatment of people involved either directly or indirectly in the incident involves a large number of agencies in a large number of tasks. Some of these are summarised in Table 2.1.

Table 2.1. Some tasks and the agencies involved

Task	Agencies
Care of the uninjured survivor	Police
	Social Services
Care of the injured	Police
	Fire
	Ambulance and Medical
Dealing with fatalities	Police
	Medical
	HM Coroner
Running the casualty bureau	Police
Dealing with friends and relatives	Police
	Medical
	Social Services
	Local Authority
Evacuation and providing shelter	Police
	Local Authority
Social and psychological support	Social Services
Religious and cultural needs	Spiritual advisers

Even this relatively small part of the overall response to a major incident can be seen to involve many more people than just the casualties, and many more agencies than just the Ambulance and Medical Services. Not surprisingly much guidance on the delivery of an adequate response has been written.

GUIDANCE

The important current guidance that has been issued to the emergency services and other agencies involved in a major incident response is listed in Table 2.2.

HEALTH SERVICE GUIDANCE

As listed above the guidance for the NHS response to a major incident is contained in *Emergency planning in the NHS: health services arrangements for dealing with major incidents*. This was initially issued in 1990 as an accompaniment to HC(90)25. This Health Circular has subsequently been superseded by HSG(93)24 but the guidance itself has not been updated.

HSG(93)24

This short guidance note sets out the context in which the main document should be read. It is made quite clear that Health Service plans should encompass not only the standard mass casualty incident, but also those arising because of food contamination, chemical or radiation hazards, and those that are transport linked. It is particularly

Table 2.2 Important guidance documents

Service	Guidance	Date
Police	*Emergency procedures manual*	1991
Fire	*Major incident emergency procedures manual*	1991
Ambulance	*Ambulance service operational arrangements: civil emergencies*	1990
NHS	*Emergency planning in the NHS: health services arrangements for dealing with accidents involving radioactivity*	1989
	Emergency planning in the NHS: health services arrangements for dealing with major incidents	1990
	Deaths in major disasters: the pathologist's role—HC90(38)	1990
Local Authority	*Emergency planning guidance to local authorities*	

concerned that contracts are put in place both between Purchasers of care and Provider Units.

District Health Authorities are specifically meant to ensure that the Ambulance Service has a leading operational role, that major hospitals develop, test, and evaluate their plans, and that funds are made available for testing and evaluating plans.

The Department of Health itself has the task of revising and keeping the handbook of guidance up to date; convening conferences of planners from hospitals, Ambulance Services, and health authorities to ensure that lessons are learned and applied; and continuing to provide funding to cover the costs of emergency planning.

Contents of the Health Service guidance

The Health Service guidance itself is set out in nine chapters, with the chapter headings shown in Box 2.2.

Key aspects of this guidance are discussed further below.

Box 2.2. Health Service guidance—contents

Glossary
General principles
Communications
Ambulance service operational arrangements
Hospital service operational requirements
Civil defence and the NHS
Local Authorities' peacetime emergencies
Health Service arrangements for dealing with accidents involving radioactivity
Health Service arrangements for dealing with chemical incidents

---

General principles

The idea of emergency planning is to ensure that the response to a major incident is effective. It is recommended that an "all hazards approach" to emergency planning is used.

Specific hazards should, however, not be ignored and known high risk sites (airports, sports stadia, and industrial complexes) should be individually assessed so that an effective response can be mounted.

> **An all hazards approach to emergency planning is recommended**

Equipment should be standardised between Ambulance and Medical Services, and with other emergency providers. Liaison is essential both within and beyond the emergency services.

Training is specifically mentioned in this part of the guidance as follows: "that health staff must receive training to prepare them for their role in a major incident and have an opportunity to practise procedures, and become familiar with the equipment (including that used in communications) and the staff with whom they will be working."

> **Training is an essential element of major incident preparedness**

It is also recommended that practical and table top exercises are held regularly and that these should test both within hospital and out of hospital plans. Full scale interservice practical exercises are recommended to take place not less than once every two years.

Communication

This section notes that good communications are essential during a major incident response. The responsibility for planning and coordination of communications within the NHS is vested in the Ambulance Service, who must provide both on site and off site communications. Off site responsibility includes communication with vehicles transporting patients and with the receiving hospitals. Communications within hospitals are the responsibility of the hospital management.

Standardisation in the method of alert is recommended so as to avoid confusion about required responses (see Chapter 3).

Specific guidance is given about alerting hospitals using ex-directory telephones, and then subsequent staff being called using cascade methods.

It is recommended that every hospital should have a *Hospital Information Centre* for collation of data about casualties and to act as a focus for communication with the police casualty bureau.

> **A Hospital Information Centre should be established**

Again, specific points are made about training and it is recommended that all personnel should be trained in the use of equipment that they may need in a major incident response.

Ambulance Service operational arrangements

This section deals with the role of the Ambulance Service during a major incident response. The key elements of this response are shown in Box 2.3.

For further guidance the reader is referred to *Ambulance service operational arrangements: civil emergencies*.

Hospital response

All listed hospitals (defined as hospitals that are adequately equipped to receive casualties on a 24 hour basis and able to provide, when needed, the Medical Incident Officer and/or a Mobile Medical and Nursing Team) are required to produce a Major Incident Plan.

> **Box 2.3.** Ambulance Service tasks
>
> Ambulances with specialised equipment immediately respond to the scene
> Additional resources are mobilised if needed for Major Incident response
> Additional resources are mobilised to maintain local emergency cover
> Medical support is transported to the scene
> Ambulance controls establish a back up facility
> Communications are provided for on site and off site communications
> Receiving hospitals are alerted as soon as possible

All listed hospitals must have a Major Incident Plan

In addition, each member of staff involved in the Major Incident Plan should have quick access to an *action card* listing his individual responsibilities, the name and telephone numbers of his key contacts, and a checklist of tasks.

All staff involved in the response should have action cards

The alerting procedures are reiterated and the roles of out of hospital responding staff (the Medical Incident Officer and the Mobile Medical Team) and their equipment are restated. Certain key areas of planning are highlighted—in particular: the existence of a Hospital Coordination Team consisting of Senior Manager, Senior Doctor, and Senior Nurse; the maintenance of communications; the setting up of a Hospital Information Centre for collation of data about casualties; the setting up of separate facilities for relatives; the adequacy of plans for dealing with the media; and other general points such as signs, identification of casualties, care of children, and debriefing. The hospital response is dealt with in detail in Chapter 15.

REGIONAL AND NATIONAL VARIATIONS

Guidance can vary from region to region and country to country. Planners should ensure that they use the most appropriate and most up to date that is available. As an example the variations current in Scotland are shown in Box 2.4.

Box 2.4. Emergency planning in Scotland

Planning

1 Guidance for the Health Service's response to a major incident in Scotland comes from a separate document entitled *Emergency planning guidance to the health service in Scotland*
2 The responsibility for planning is devolved to each Health Board of which there are 15 in Scotland. Each Health Board has an Emergency Planning Officer. The varying geography and population densities necessitate different arrangements throughout the country, and Emergency Planning Officers should be contacted to find out the local arrangements

On site arrangements and terminology

1 The terms "Gold," "Silver," and "Bronze" are not used
2 The term "Nursing Incident Officer" is not used
3 There has been a recommendation that red should be the predominant colour of clothing worn by doctors and nurses at the scene
4 Mobile Medical Teams are only to be despatched if requested by the Site Medical Officer or, before his arrival, the Ambulance Incident Officer
5 The place of the coroner in England is fulfilled by the Procurator Fiscal in Scotland

The Ambulance Service

1 There is only one Ambulance Service in Scotland—the Scottish Ambulance Service. It has 477 emergency vehicles all of which contain similar equipment. In addition there are Mobile Ambulance Control Vehicles (MACVs) and Emergency Support Units (ESUs) dotted throughout the country. All MACVs and ESUs contain standardised equipment. The District Ambulance Officer's Vehicle would be used as the Ambulance Control until the MACV arrives. Control vehicles do not use green lights
2 There is no Emergency Reserve Channel in Scotland
3 Plans do not include the provision of an Ambulance Safety Officer

---

Summary
- The Health Service's response for a major incident should be part of a combined response
- Specific guidance exists regarding the nature of the Health Services' response
- Key elements of guidance include all risk planning and adequacy of training

3

Outline response

This chapter will answer the following questions:

- How is a major incident declared?
- What are the initial response and actions of the emergency services?
- What is the initial response at the hospital?

DECLARING A MAJOR INCIDENT

Each emergency service and every listed hospital will have a Major Incident Plan which allows the rapid mobilisation of additional resources. The problem is often not the enforcement of the Plan, but rather a reluctance to institute it. This may be for reasons of professional pride, for fear of criticism of calling a major incident unnecessarily, or out of ignorance. None of these is acceptable. If in any doubt a major incident should be declared.

At the hospital confusion may arise unless there is a clear message from the scene that a major incident has been declared and the hospital Major Incident Plan is to be put into action. For this reason the notifying messages to the hospital have been standardised:

---

1 *Major incident—standby*
   This alerts the hospital that a major incident is possibly imminent. A limited number of staff need to be informed
2 *Major incident declared—activate plan*
   In this case the incident has occurred and a full response is required

   Either of these orders can be rescinded at any time by the order:
3 *Major incident—cancelled*

If it is not possible to give a clear message to the hospital, casualties may arrive when no extra provision has been made. In such cases the hospital should activate its own plan internally.

The orders will be initiated at the scene and relayed to the hospital via ambulance control, preferably directly to the hospital switchboard. Should the message be given directly to the emergency department, it is important that this is immediately relayed to the switchboard so that the process of alerting key personnel can start.

EMERGENCY SERVICES

The initial response of the emergency services depends to a large extent on the quality of the information they receive, and its source. It is not the routine policy of the Ambulance Service to dispatch multiple vehicles until it has been independently confirmed that there are multiple casualties. The Fire Service, however, will dispatch a graded number of vehicles as a result of the initial information, depending on the perceived need—a so called "predetermined attendance."

At the scene of the incident the first priorities for each emergency service are to save life, to gain control, to gather and relay information, and to ensure that an adequate response is made. The initial objectives are therefore common to each emergency service as are their overall aims, which are summarised in Box 3.1.

Box 3.1. The common objectives of the emergency services

Save life
Prevent escalation of the incident
Relieve suffering
Protect the environment
Protect property
Rapidly restore normality
Assist any criminal investigation or enquiry

As an illustration, the build up of emergency services and the declaration of a major incident at the scene of the King's Cross Underground fire on 18 November 1987 are shown in Table 3.1.

COMMAND STRUCTURE

The first member of each emergency service at the scene will become the *Incident Officer*. It is usual for the job of Incident Officer to be handed over to more senior ranks as they arrive. The Incident Officer is identified by a distinctive chequered tabard (Box 3.2).

Box 3.2. Incident Officer tabards

Incident Officer	**Tabard colours**
Police	Blue and white
Fire	Red and white
Ambulance	Green and white

The Incident Officer is an administrator and will not be directly involved in casualty rescue or treatment. Those officers who are controlling work at the "coal face" are termed BRONZE (operational) control. Each is responsible to his own Incident Officer, with the Incident Officers collectively forming SILVER (tactical) control. Silver (tactical) control is not static as the Incident Officers will move about the scene, including walking into the Bronze (operational) area. GOLD (strategic) control will be some distance

Table 3.1. Emergency service response to a major incident

	London Fire Brigade	Metropolitan Police	London Ambulance Service
Time			
19:30	Escalator fire		
19:34	Summoned		
19:35		Local division alerted	
19:41		New Scotland Yard central command alerted	
19:42– 19:46	PDA arrives (Four pumps + turntable ladder + forward control unit)		
19:44	Four more pumps requested		
19:45		Inspector in car forms police FCU; requests ambulances	
19:47			Ambulance control alerted
19:49	Four more pumps requested Four ambulances requested		
19:57			First ambulance on scene
20:00			Second ambulance on scene
20:01		Traffic motor cycles deployed	
20:08			Two hospitals on "STANDBY"
20:12		More ambulances requested	
20:13		Major incident box sent from Holborn station to University College Hospital	
20:16			Major incident "DECLARED"
20:15– 20:41	Eight more pumps requested		Ambulances arrive (total = 14)
20:16– 21:32			
20:20		FCU becomes RVP for MMTs; helicopter transfers medical supplies between hospitals	
20:41	Ten more pumps requested		
21:00		>100 officers on scene	
21:48	"Fire surrounded" (controlled)		
22:09			Emergency Control Vehicle arrives on scene

Prepared from the Department of Transport Report: Investigation into the King's Cross Underground Fire.
PDA, predetermined attendance; FCU, Forward Control Unit; RVP, rendezvous point; MMT, Mobile Medical Team.

from the scene and comprises senior officers of the emergency services, together with representatives from the Local Authority and other involved agencies (for example, the military). This principle of the tiered command is illustrated in Figure 3.1. Scene command and control is discussed in detail in Chapter 12.

The first emergency vehicle of each service at the scene will become the *Forward Control Unit*, until the official control vehicle arrives. The Forward Control Unit will act as a marshalling point for further personnel and should be the only vehicle of each service that does not extinguish its rotating beacons, therefore enabling it to be easily identified.

The doctor in command at the scene is known as the *Medical Incident Officer* (MIO). The doctor in command at Bronze (operational) control—who is the eyes and ears of the Medical Incident Officer—is known as the *Forward Medical Incident Officer* (FMIO), and liaises directly with the Forward Ambulance Incident Officer (FAIO).

Doctors and nurses who are deployed from hospitals will form *Mobile Medical Teams* (MMTs). All members of these teams must report to the MIO for tasking on arrival at the scene—they will only take orders from the MIO or his deputy, unless it is a safety instruction. Individual *Immediate Care Doctors* can be mobilised where a local scheme exists. These doctors are also responsible to the MIO. Discipline among members of

21

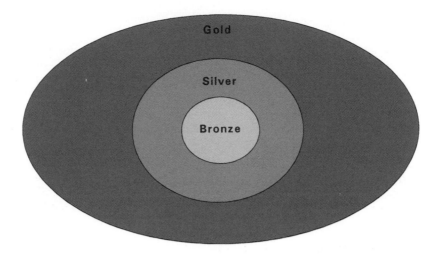

Figure 3.1 The levels of control at a major incident. Note: this represents a *concept* rather than physical barriers. Although there is a cordon around the Silver area, there is none to encompass the Gold area and there may be none around the Bronze area. There may be any number of Bronze areas within the overall incident (Silver area).

the medical teams and individual doctors is paramount, if control of medical resources is to be maintained. This can be difficult to achieve where senior medical staff who are used to working autonomously are unwilling to accept orders, or the Incident Officer lacks the training to command authoritatively. The Health Service command and control is discussed in detail in Chapter 13.

Discipline of medical staff is essential to maintaining control

Communications

Good communications are vital at a major incident (see Chapter 11); this is especially so in the early phase, and guarantees a prompt and appropriate response from each emergency service.

The Police, Fire, and Ambulance Services will park their Forward Control Units in close proximity to each other and communications between the three units should be established.

The quality of the first information that is passed from the scene will be important in determining the speed and adequacy of the subsequent response. The acronym ETHANE is recommended as a reminder of the key points (Table 3.2).

Table 3.2. Initial information to be passed from the scene of a major incident

E	Exact location	Grid reference
T	Type of incident	Rail, chemical, road
H	Hazards	Current and potential
A	Access	From which direction to approach
N	Number of casualties	And their severity/type
E	Emergency services	Present and required

The Police

The Police are in overall control of the incident. Their role is to secure the scene and facilitate the other emergency services. The officer in charge of the scene is the Senior Police Officer, regardless of his or her rank. In some circumstances the Senior Fire Officer will assume control of the Bronze (operational) area of the scene if there is a specific hazard, and will remain in control until that hazard has been contained.

> **The Police have precedence over other emergency services at the scene of a major incident**

The initial responsibilities of the Police are listed in Box 3.3.

Box 3.3. Initial responsibilities of the Police

Command of the incident and establishment of a forward control
Saving of life
Prevention or escalation of the incident
Evacuation of those still in danger
Activation of other emergency services
Provision of traffic control
Liaison with and facilitation of the other emergency services
Maintenance of records of the casualties
Identification of the dead
Maintenance of public order
Protection of the environment and property
Criminal investigation and assistance with official enquiries
Liaison with the media

The scene of a major incident should always be treated as a scene of crime (unless it is a natural disaster—see Chapter 1). Medical staff have a responsibility to preserve evidence by limiting their interference with the scene. In the case of the dead, the Police will act as Her Majesty's Coroner's representative. The Coroner has a legal obligation to investigate the cause of death resulting from the incident.

The Police will assist the initial enquiries of specialist accident investigation bodies, such as the Air Accident Investigation Branch in aviation incidents. Additionally, they will coordinate the movements of the media, who may arrive very quickly, and will provide them with early, regular press releases.

The Fire Service

The Fire Service have a responsibility to contain and eliminate any hazards at the scene, and to rescue people who are trapped in the wreckage or in a hazardous environment. The immediate area around the incident will be under the control of the Senior Fire Officer until such hazards have been neutralised. Specific hazards include:

- Fire
- Chemical spillage
- Electricity (for example, rail incident)
- Risk of explosion

23

- Flooding
- Nuclear material.

The initial responsibilities of the Fire Service are listed in Box 3.4.

Box 3.4. Initial responsibilities of the Fire Service

Establishment of a forward control
Saving of life
Prevention of escalation of the incident
Fire fighting
Elimination of hazards
Rescue of entrapped casualties
Clearance of routes in and out of the wreckage
Liaison with the other emergency services
Provision of specialist equipment (lighting, lifting, tentage)
Freeing of the dead

The Ambulance Service

The role of the Ambulance Service is to assess, treat, and transport the injured. The Ambulance Incident Officer will request a number of ambulances determined by an initial appraisal. It is important that the officer on the ground declares a major incident as soon as it is evident, and does not rely on ambulance control to deduce this.

On declaring a major incident ambulance control will activate the emergency reserve channel (ERC). Vehicles that are not allocated to the major incident response can continue to operate on their normal channel. An Emergency Control Vehicle (ECV) is despatched to the scene to provide on site communications (see Chapter 11); a senior officer will also be sent to assume the role of Ambulance Incident Officer. Other emergency service control rooms are contacted to ensure that they have responded. Hospitals are alerted and will be told to "activate plan" (first receiving hospitals) or to "stand by." An urgent bedstate should be obtained to help plan the distribution of casualties. Immediate care doctors should be mobilised if available locally, and a Medical Incident Officer and Mobile Medical Team(s) are requested from hospital. An Ambulance Liaison Officer will be sent to the hospital emergency department to help with communications between the hospital, ambulance control, and the scene.

Additional resources can be obtained from neighbouring Health Authorities or by considering the use of voluntary services (St John's Ambulance, British Red Cross—see Chapter 8).

The initial responsibilities of the Ambulance Service are listed in Box 3.5.

THE MEDICAL SERVICES

Hospital

When a major incident "activate plan" message is received, the immediate actions of the hospital can be considered in terms of:

- Preparation of the hospital
- Call in of key staff
- Nomination and dispatch of a Medical Incident Officer and/or Mobile Medical Team as requested.

> **Box 3.5.** Initial responsibilities of the Ambulance Service
>
> Establishment of a forward control
> Saving of life
> Prevention of further injury
> Relief of suffering
> Liaison with other emergency services
> Determination of the receiving hospitals
> Mobilisation of necessary additional medical services
> Provision of a Casualty Clearing Station
> Provision of an ambulance parking and loading point
> Documentation of the movement of casualties to hospital

Subsequently the hospital must receive, triage, and treat casualties as they arrive.

A *Hospital Information Centre* is set up for internal use and will collate information relating to availability of operating rooms (theatres), bed occupancy, casualty data (for example, listing their condition as satisfactory, seriously ill, or critically ill), and whether relatives have been informed. This centre will work closely with the *Police Casualty Documentation Team* (usually stationed in the emergency department) who will report to the Casualty Bureau. This information can be used to answer relatives' enquiries.

Staff must be aware of the chain of command, which will be different to normal working practice. The hospital response services are discussed in more detail in Chapter 15.

Pre-hospital

The detailed roles of the Medical and Nursing Incident Officers are discussed in Chapter 13. The detailed role of the Mobile Medical Team is discussed in Chapter 14. The key responsibilities of the Medical Incident Officer, Nursing Incident Officer, and Mobile Medical Team are listed in Boxes 3.6–3.8.

> **Box 3.6.** Responsibilities of the Medical Incident Officer
>
> Coordination of medical resources at the scene
> Provision of adequate personnel to save life, to prevent further injury, and to relieve suffering
> Liaison with other emergency services
> Communication of necessary information to the receiving hospital
> Establishment of a Casualty Clearing Station
> Monitoring of triage and treatment at the scene
> Ensuring that adequate documentation of injuries and treatment given
> Ensuring that casualties are evacuated to the most appropriate hospital
> Organisation of relief medical staff and recognition of individual fatigue
> Provision of staff to pronounce death

> **Box 3.7.** Responsibilities of the Nursing Incident Officer
>
> Liaison with the MIO and AIO
> Determination of the most appropriate duties for individual nurses
> Supervision of triage and treatment performed by nurses
> Collation of casualty numbers and their injuries/triage priorities
> Allocation of controlled drugs to nursing staff
> Monitoring of the welfare of all nursing staff present

> **Box 3.8.** Responsibilities of the Mobile Medical Team
>
> Life saving treatment and relief of suffering
> Prevention of further injury to patients

OTHER AGENCIES

Agencies other than the Police, Fire, Ambulance, and Medical Services may be involved in the initial response to a major incident. These can include the following:

- The Local Authority
- The military
- Volunteer organisations
- HM Coastguard—for civil maritime search and rescue
- Industry—to provide specialist equipment or knowledge
- Central Government.

More details are given in Chapter 8.

Summary
- Standardised alert messages will ensure a consistent hospital response
- The Police are in overall command at the scene. The emergency services' command structure is tiered
- Emergency services have a combined response
- Within the combined response each service has specific responsibilities
- The response at the hospital is controlled by the Hospital Coordination Team

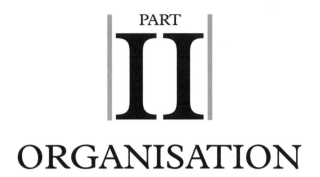

PART

II

ORGANISATION

CHAPTER

4

The medical services

After reading this chapter you should be able to answer the following questions:

- How are the medical services organised on a day to day basis?
- How should the hospital medical services be organised during a major incident?
- How are medical services organised at the scene of a major incident?

INTRODUCTION

The medical services in the United Kingdom have recently undergone a complete reorganisation. This has affected all aspects of health care delivery, and the major incident response is no exception. It is important to understand the new structure of the service if effective planning is to take place.

The service is now managed by the National Health Service Executive (NHSE). Eight regional outposts of the NHSE are currently being set up to monitor the provision of care. Care is bought by purchasers who may either be general practitioners or Commissioners acting either individually or as consortia. Care is delivered by provider units who hold contracts with purchasers. This structure is summarised in Figure 4.1.

Emergency care (which includes the major incident response) is an integral part of the contract at the individual provider level. The contracting process needs to ensure that major incident provision is seamless (that is, that the cover is complete and does not stop and start as artificial boundaries of responsibility are crossed). The new Health Service, with its plethora of providers each driven by contracts, makes this much more difficult to achieve.

Almost all provider units (including ambulance services) are NHS Trusts. The typical management structure of a trust is summarised in Figure 4.2.

The management structure of individual trusts is of course the responsibility of each trust, and many variations will therefore exist. Whatever the organisation of a particular trust, it is unlikely that it will be able to manage a major incident response unchanged. Trusts have been designed to manage contracts, activity, and finance rather than emergency clinical situations. Some services and teams do, however, manage emergencies on a daily basis and the expertise for management of a major incident should be available.

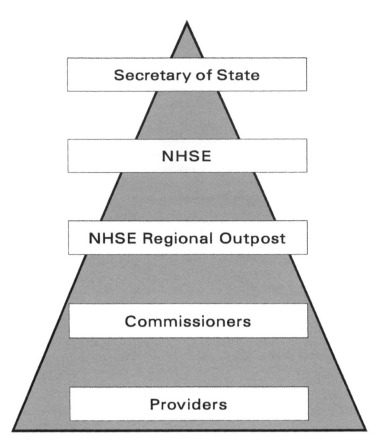

Figure 4.1. National Health Service management organisation

The structure of the Health Service makes seamlessness difficult to achieve

Planning is a vital part of the preparedness of a provider unit for a major incident, and the key element of planning should be the setting up of the command and control elements of the response. The success of Major Incident Plans depends largely on good control. The ability of the staff to treat casualties is not usually in question.

MANAGEMENT OF THE HOSPITAL RESPONSE

This is dealt with in more detail in Chapter 15. Once an incident has been declared, the day to day organisation of the hospital service needs to be changed to cope with the influx of casualties. Efficient structures must be put in place both to control the overall hospital response and to ensure that the extraordinary demands placed on specific areas (such as reception and surgery) can be met.

Once the major incident procedure has been activated, the hospital response is managed by the *Hospital Coordination Team*. The team consists of a Medical Coordinator (usually the Medical Director or deputy) who is in charge, with a Senior Manager, a Senior Nurse, and a Senior Emergency Physician (usually the consultant in charge of major incident planning or deputy) assisting. Each of these assistants will have his or her area of responsibility—the manager ensuring optimum support services, the nurse ensuring that the hospital is prepared, and the emergency physician organising the reception areas. As the response progresses the team coordinates the various staff and resources, and eventually returns the unit to normal working.

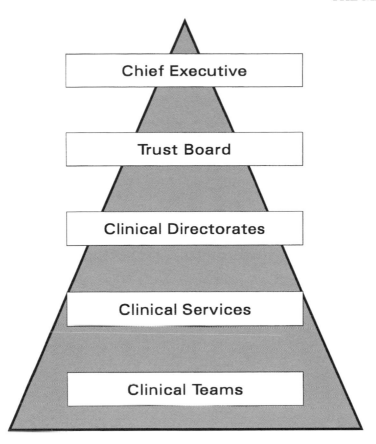

Figure 4.2. Management within an NHS trust

Reception of casualties

This is a vital part of the response and is usually the most chaotic. The Chief Triage Officer retriages the patients as they arrive, and assigns them to the various parts of the reception area according to their priority. The Surgical Triage Officer (usually the Duty Consultant Surgeon) and the Medical Triage Officer (usually either the Duty Consultant Physician or the Duty Consultant from the intensive care unit) supervise both the clinical activity and the allocation of priorities for further treatment and surgery. The Team Coordinator forms the medical and nursing staff into treatment and transfer teams, and allocates them to clinical areas as requested.

Surgical response

The surgical response can be especially difficult to organise because the casualties may be in a number of different areas. It is essential that triage decisions for surgery are all taken by one person (the Surgical Triage Officer), and that the information on which these decisions are based is accurate. To this end the senior surgeons in other surgical areas must be in regular contact with the Surgical Triage Officer.

Priority setting in the surgical area involves not only the ordering of patients for surgery, but also the ordering of procedures for individual patients. It is essential that surgery is kept to the minimum necessary to save life and limb while operating time is at a premium. This aspect of control is difficult because it differs from normal clinical practice.

MANAGEMENT OF THE OUT OF HOSPITAL RESPONSE

This is dealt with in some detail in Chapter 13. The medical response must be closely coordinated with that of the ambulance service, and to that end it is essential that the Medical and Ambulance Incident Officers liaise frequently.

The provision of medical personnel on scene usually takes some time and all the command and control positions shown may not be filled (Figure 4.3). Those sent to the scene must be prepared to fill these positions if necessary, even if it means not giving medical support to the casualties. As with the hospital response high quality management at the scene is essential if the best outcome is to be achieved.

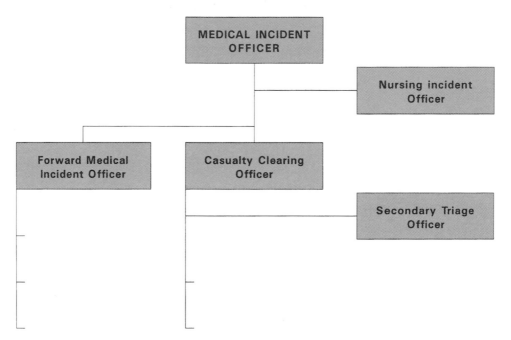

Figure 4.3. Medical organisation at the scene

Summary
- The health service is contract based with a purchaser provider split
- It is more difficult to achieve a seamless major incident response under such circumstances
- The structure of trusts is variable
- The hospital major incident response is controlled by the Hospital Coordination Team
- The reception and surgical triage of casualties in hospital require proper coordination
- The out of hospital response is controlled by the Ambulance and Medical Incident Officers

5

The Ambulance Service

After reading this chapter you should be able to answer the following questions:

- What is the organisation and rank structure of the Ambulance Service?
- What is the role of the Ambulance Service in a major incident?
- How can the medical services assist the Ambulance Service at a major incident?

ORGANISATION

Ambulance personnel are, on the whole, trained to work in pairs to give care to a single patient, with each crew operating independently but tasked by a central ambulance control. In day to day operations the crew will act on their own initiative without the supervision of an ambulance officer, one taking the role of attendant (directing patient care) and the other being responsible for driving. It is the current aim to ensure that one of the two person crew on every frontline ambulance is trained as a "paramedic."

At the scene of a major incident it can therefore be anticipated that up to half of the personnel who attend the scene in frontline ambulances will have paramedical skills.

RANK STRUCTURE

The rank structure of the Ambulance Services in the United Kingdom is not consistent and the traditional ranks of this uniformed service have to a large extent been replaced with managerial appointments (for example, "Chief Executive" replacing "Chief Ambulance Officer"), reflecting the change to Ambulance Service Trusts (Figures 5.1 and 5.2).

In addition to their rank ambulance personnel will identify themselves as either a *technician* or a *paramedic*. The paramedic will have extended skills including endotracheal intubation and intravenous cannulation, and should therefore be tasked to work in appropriate areas at the scene.

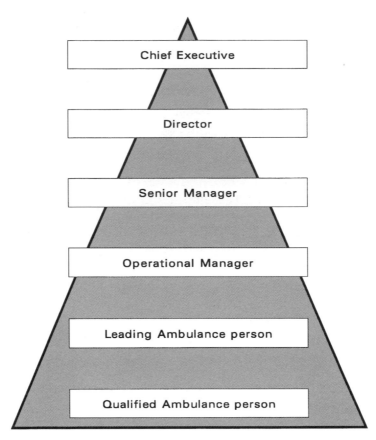

Figure 5.1. Rank structure of an Ambulance Service Trust

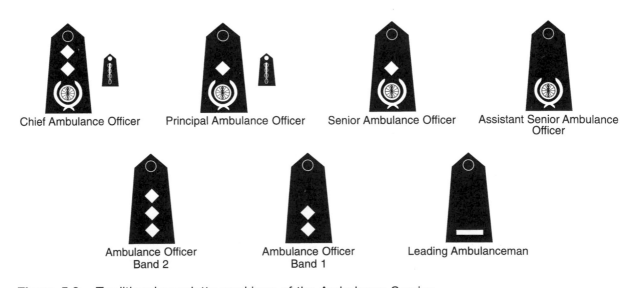

Figure 5.2. Traditional epaulette markings of the Ambulance Service

Identify those with extended skills and ensure that they work in appropriate areas

AMBULANCE SERVICE ROLE IN A MAJOR INCIDENT

Action of the first crew on scene

The actions of the crew of the first ambulance on the scene of a major incident are critical in determining the speed of mobilisation of further ambulance and medical resources, and of ensuring that the hospitals are given the maximum possible time to prepare for receiving multiple casualties. In this phase of the response, time is life—a delay in declaring a major incident or an inadequate response will cost lives.

The ambulance *attendant* will assume the role of the Ambulance Incident Officer; this role will be handed over to a more senior officer on his or her arrival. The *driver* will stay with the vehicle and maintain communications with the vehicle and with Central Control. Under no circumstances should this crew become involved in patient treatment because this will remove their ability to provide liaison with other services, to assess the scene as a whole, and to provide a continuous conduit of information as the incident develops. The driver should contact Control and report their arrival. He will give the location of the incident and may give a brief visual description, but the first substantial situation report will come from the attendant after a rapid scene reconnaissance. The information that should be contained in this report is given in Table 5.1.

Table 5.1. Initial information to be passed from the scene of a major incident

E	Exact location	Grid reference
T	Type of incident	Rail, chemical, road
H	Hazards	Current and potential
A	Access	From which direction to approach
N	Number of casualties	And their severity/type
E	Emergency services	Present and required

Most importantly, the term "major incident" must be used as early as possible in the radio message to Central Control. It may be difficult to make the distinction between a *potential* and an *actual* major incident in the first few minutes, especially if the number of casualties cannot be easily assessed. Box 5.1 is a sample initial situation report from the first ambulance at the scene to Central Control.

Box 5.1.	First radio situation report
Mobile:	**Major incident standby** timed at 16:15 hours. Acknowledge major incident standby, over.
Control:	Major incident standby, over.
Mobile:	Yes. Location is level crossing one mile west of Markham village, grid figures one-seven-eight two-two-zero. Passenger train derailment. Fire and electricity hazards. Access from road Alpha three-two approaching through Markham. Estimated up to fifty, five-zero, casualties. Request fire and police attendance, acknowledge over.

As soon as it is evident that there is a definite major incident, the attendant must pass the message, "Major incident declared" (Box 5.2).

The first ambulance at the scene will become the Forward Ambulance Control Unit and the rendezvous point for all Health Service resources arriving at the scene. It should therefore be the only ambulance vehicle which does not extinguish its blue beacon. The role of this vehicle as the Ambulance Service incident control and rendezvous point will be taken over by the Emergency Control Vehicle or "ECV" (a mobile communications centre) when this arrives—the ECV may have a blue *or* green beacon.

Box 5.2. Declaring a major incident

Mobile: **Major incident declared** at 16:18 hours. Confirm excess of one hundred figures one-zero-zero casualties, acknowledge major incident declared, over.

Control: Major incident declared. Out.

The actions of the first crew on the scene are summarised in Box 5.3. As stated the attendant will start to set up a Casualty Clearing Station. At this early phase of the incident this may involve no more than identifying an area where the walking wounded and uninjured survivors should gather and wait.

Box 5.3. The actions of the first ambulance crew

Driver
- Parks as near to the scene as safety permits
- Leaves the roof beacon on (indicating the vehicle is acting as the ambulance control point)
- Confirms arrival at scene with Ambulance Control
- Maintains communications with the attendant
- Stays with the vehicle until instructed by a senior ambulance officer
- Leaves the ignition keys

Attendant
- Carries out scene reconnaissance
- Gives a situation report to Control
- Declares a major incident
- Selects location of the ambulance parking point
- Decides the need for medical teams or special equipment
- Sets up key areas: control point, parking point, Casualty Clearing Station

---

Actions of Central Ambulance Control

On receipt of a message at Central Ambulance Control warning of or declaring a major incident, the duty controllers will refer to their action cards. There are two primary tasks, which are to coordinate the response of Ambulance Service vehicles to the scene and to ensure that all necessary organisations and individuals have been informed. These tasks will be considered for a "major incident standby" and "major incident declared."

Major incident—standby

Controller 1—This controller will log the initial information from the scene and inform the remaining control staff, before despatching the first vehicles. The timings of all subsequent actions must be logged. Personnel en route may be advised to refer to their action cards and to dress appropriately. The nearest Senior Manager will be sent to the scene to take over the role of Ambulance Incident Officer from the first responding ambulanceman. Radio communications will be switched to the Emergency Reserve Channel and all call signs informed immediately before this occurs. An Emergency Control Vehicle (for scene control and communications) and an Emergency Support Unit (with medical supplies) are dispatched to the scene. Control staff going off duty are held back and ambulance officers who will fill key roles at the scene are alerted.

Controller 2—The Police and Fire Control rooms are advised of the situation, under a reciprocal arrangement. The nearest local listed hospital(s) are informed through dedicated lines to the hospital switchboard (or directly via the Accident and Emergency Departments). Senior Ambulance Officers are alerted (Chief Executive; Directors [Operations and Communications]; Senior Manager in charge of communications) as are the Emergency Planning Officer and adjoining ambulance controls.

Major incident declared—activate plan

Controller 1—Further ambulances are sent to the scene along with officers to administer the following areas: Ambulance Parking Point, Ambulance Loading Point, and Casualty Clearing Station. In addition, an Ambulance Liaison Officer is needed in each of the receiving hospitals to provide communications with Control. Personnel en route are informed of the change in status of the incident, the best approach, and the location of the rendezvous point. Transport, if required, is organised for the Medical Incident Officer and Mobile Medical Team(s). Communications are confirmed with the control vehicle at the scene and the receiving hospitals. Patient transport vehicles (minibus ambulances) may also be redeployed if necessary.

Controller 2—Receiving hospitals are informed that the Major Incident is declared and the plan should be activated. Ambulance controls in adjacent authorities are advised that there is a major incident and the level of available resources is established; these are requested if necessary. Off duty staff are called in, perhaps using a cascade system and sometimes with the assistance of a local radio/TV broadcast. The Voluntary Aid societies are informed and given a rendezvous point; the Police should be told that these societies have been requested. The Blood Transfusion Service is contacted.

The Central Ambulance Control will be managed by a Senior Control Manager during this period. His primary role is to liaise with the Ambulance Incident Officer (AIO) and provide the required resources and equipment for the scene; he will ensure that the control tasks listed above are completed and in addition will do the following:

- Ensure completion of all documents in relation to the incident along with tape recordings of the associated communications
- On extended incidents ensure that control staff receive adequate rest breaks
- Advise all Health Service agencies of the official "stand down" from the incident.

Ambulance Service responsibilities at the scene

The responsibilities of the Ambulance Service at the scene are listed in Box 5.4.

The objectives of the Ambulance Service are clearly to provide the best possible care for the injured at the scene, and to arrange expeditious transport of the right patient to the right hospital. Ambulance Control will have information regarding which hospitals can provide a Medical Incident Officer, Mobile Medical Team, and receive casualties on a 24 hour basis—the "listed" hospital. Those hospitals to which the AIO sends casualties are the "receiving" hospitals. In England and Wales it is the Ambulance Service who have the responsibility to select these hospitals. The Medical Incident Officer (MIO) may have local knowledge about the appropriateness of hospitals for individual casualties, and advises the AIO about this. It is not the MIO's responsibility to decide *where* the Mobile Medical Team(s) should come from, only to determine the *degree* of response needed at the scene.

The management of the scene in terms of deployment of ambulance personnel around the scene is discussed in Chapter 13.

Box 5.4. Responsibilities of the Ambulance Service at the scene

Establishment of a forward control
Saving of life
Prevention of further injury
Relief of suffering
Liaison with other emergency services
Determination of the receiving hospitals
Mobilisation of necessary additional medical services
Provision of communications for NHS resources at the scene
Provision of a Casualty Clearing Station
Provision of an ambulance parking and loading point
Determination of priorities for treatment and evacuation (triage)
Arrangement of means of transporting the injured
Documentation of the movement of casualties

MEDICAL AID TO THE AMBULANCE SERVICE

The Ambulance Service has a statutory duty to provide medical care to the injured and to transport them to hospital. There is much the Medical Services can do, however, to support the Ambulance Service in pre-hospital casualty treatment, and this is particularly so in the case of a major incident. The areas in which the Medical Services can supplement the Ambulance Service's role are shown in Box 5.5.

Box 5.5. Medical aid to the Ambulance Service
- Experienced clinicians to perform the triage sort
- Additional personnel to perform advanced airway manoeuvres (for example, intubation) and obtain venous access
- The surgical management of the airway (cricothyrotomy) and life threatening chest injury (needle and tube thoracostomy)
- The extended management of hypovolaemia, when the paramedic's protocol is exhausted, including the prescription of blood
- The administration of analgesic drugs
- The administration of local and general anaesthesia
- Emergency surgical procedures to facilitate extrication (for example, amputation)
- Advice from the MIO regarding the best disposal of individual patients
- Nursing staff to provide "care" for the patients delayed at the scene, beyond simple treatment of their injuries

Summary
- The first ambulance crew on scene will not be involved in patient treatment, but will form the Forward Ambulance Control Unit
- A major incident must be declared early
- The skills of individual personnel should be recognised and used appropriately
- The Medical Services can provide considerable aid to the Ambulance Service at the scene

CHAPTER

6

The Police

After reading this chapter you should be able to answer these questions:

- What is the organisation and rank structure of the Police?
- What is the role of the Police at a major incident?
- How can the Police assist the Health Services at a major incident?

ORGANISATION

There are 52 Police forces in the United Kingdom. Most forces are responsible for a "county" area (or "region" in Scotland); in London there are two forces (Metropolitan and City), whereas in Northern Ireland policing is carried out by the Royal Ulster Constabulary. As well as these local forces there are a number of others with special responsibilities: British Transport, Ministry of Defence, Atomic Energy Authority, and Royal Parks.

RANK STRUCTURE

The rank structure of the British Police (excluding the Metropolitan Police) is as shown in Figures 6.1 and 6.2.

The Metropolitan Police (which is five to 10 times larger than the county forces) is commanded by a Commissioner aided by a deputy, some assistants, and deputy assistants. An additional rank of Commander exists above that of Chief Superintendent.

ROLE OF THE POLICE AT A MAJOR INCIDENT

The Police have precedence at the scene of a major incident—that is, they retain overall control. In the presence of a specific hazard (such as fire or chemical spillage), the Police will surrender control to the *immediate* scene area (the Bronze (operational) area) to the Senior Fire Officer.

The first Police officer on scene is responsible for establishing a forward control, for assessing the scene, and for requesting further Police and other emergency service

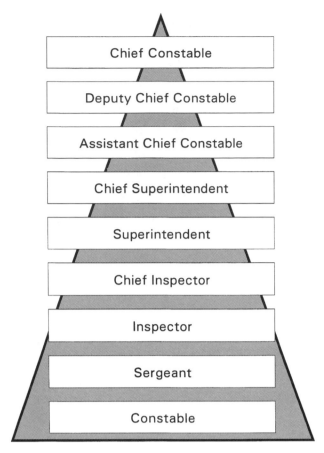

Figure 6.1. Rank structure of the British Police (excluding the Metropolitan Police)

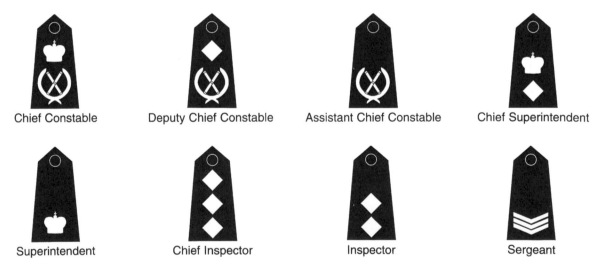

Figure 6.2. Traditional epaulette markings of the Police

resources. It is vital that the initial message contains the term "major incident," if valuable time is to be saved. The information that should be contained in the initial message is listed in Table 6.1.

Police Control has a responsibility to inform other emergency service controls when the Major Incident Plan is activated. This first officer must not be distracted and become

Table 6.1. Initial information to be passed from the scene of a major incident

E	Exact location	Grid reference
T	Type of incident	Rail, chemical, road
H	Hazards	Current and potential
A	Access	From which direction to approach
N	Number of casualties	And their severity/type
E	Emergency services	Present and required

involved in administering first aid, otherwise his ability to function as a coordinator is lost.

The initial responsibilities of the Police are given in Box 6.1.

Box 6.1. Initial responsibilities of the Police

Control of the incident and establishing a Forward Control Point
Saving of life
Prevention of escalation of the incident
Evacuation of those still in danger
Ensuring the activation of other emergency services
Provision of traffic control
Liaison with and facilitation of the other emergency services
Maintenance of records of the casualties
Identification of the dead
Maintenance of public order
Protection of the environment and property
Criminal investigation and assistance with official enquiries
Liaison with the media

Those members of the public who are in imminent danger after the incident, such as from fire, chemical exposure, or radioactive contamination, will be evacuated to safety by the Police. The Police will set up cordons around the scene, to limit public access, and will record the names of *bona fide* rescue workers on the scene; it is a Police responsibility to confirm the identity of those who claim to be qualified to give help. Medical staff must carry official identity badges: *no badge, no admittance.*

Specific roles of the Police that will be considered are the following:

- Running a Casualty Bureau
- Care of uninjured survivors
- Care of relatives and friends
- Identification and handling of the dead
- Maintenance of free traffic flow
- Supervision of volunteers
- Maintenance of public order
- Handling of the media.

Casualty Bureau

This term strictly refers to the central contact point where all information on casualties, survivors, and evacuees is collated. It is often more loosely applied to include the branches of this bureau which are set up at the receiving hospitals (and the mortuary and survivor reception centre) as *Police Documentation Teams.*

The telephone number of the Casualty Bureau is the number that will be broadcast by television and radio media to alert relatives, and provides them with a source of contact. As well as being a service to the public, this will greatly assist the Police in the identification of the dead and the seriously injured.

In the case of an airline crash, the Police may be supported by the Emergency Procedures Information Centre (EPIC) at Heathrow Airport. This is staffed by British Airways staff and will collate all those enquiries directed through the airline. This may help the Police by providing, for example, next of kin data. The number of EPIC will also be broadcast.

The functions of the Casualty Bureau are summarised in Box 6.2.

Box 6.2. Functions of the Casualty Bureau

Record the location of the injured, and their condition
Gather information on the identity of the injured and dead
Gather information on the location of survivors and evacuees
Compile a list of missing persons involved in the incident
Answer enquiries from relatives and friends relating to survivors, injured, and dead

---

The care of uninjured survivors

The Police are responsible for sheltering and feeding the uninjured survivors in the short term, and may set up a *Survivor Reception Centre*. Those who cannot return to their homes immediately will be moved to *rest centres*, and some may require longer term accommodation—these facilities will be provided by the Local Authority. All survivors must have access to medical services in these areas.

Survivors are regarded as witnesses to what often becomes a criminal enquiry. Initially, at the Survivor Reception Centre, it may be appropriate to take only names and addresses, because individuals may be too distressed to provide a full statement. The requirements for a Survivor Reception Centre are listed in Box 6.3.

Box 6.3. Requirements for a Survivor Reception Centre

Secure area away from the public and unrestricted press
Food
Water
Sanitation
Dry clothing
Medical facility for minor injuries and further triage
Police Documentation Team
Social workers (financial and psychological support)

The care of relatives and friends

Relatives and friends of the injured and dead may have been involved in the incident and form a proportion of the uninjured survivors. They must be handled with particular sensitivity.

Alternatively, relatives and friends may make their way to the incident. These people should be directed to a *Relatives' Reception Centre*. This will be located outside the outer cordon and adjacent to a rest centre, where they can be reunited with the survivors.

The dead

The confirmation of death can only be pronounced by a doctor. This should be done in the presence of a Police officer, with the time and officer's personal number noted on the appropriate label.

The identification of the dead is the responsibility of the *Police Identification Commission* and is overseen by the Police Incident Officer. The Police are responsible for informing the next of kin when the deceased has been identified.

The dead cannot be moved without the permission of HM Coroner, unless they are preventing access to the living, or unless bodies or parts of bodies are in danger of being destroyed by fire or corrosive chemicals. If bodies must be moved they should ideally be photographed first, and their original position clearly marked.

> **Do not move the dead, unless they are preventing access to the living**

When authority is granted to move a body it is the responsibility of the Police to do this. Bodies are taken to a *temporary mortuary* for forensic pathological examination and formal identification—*do not* remove rings or other valuables for safe keeping as this may hinder identification. Further discussion about the dead is given in Chapter 19.

Traffic control

The maintenance of free traffic flow and the organisation of vehicle marshalling areas ensure the continued smooth running of the incident, and are the responsibility of the Police.

Supervision of volunteers

Volunteers and voluntary organisations are often welcome at the scene of a major incident. They can provide additional pairs of hands for manual work or act as runners, thereby releasing skilled rescuers for other duties. The volunteers must be logged in and out of the scene, and carefully monitored to ensure that their actions are appropriate. The Police will provide the necessary supervision.

Welfare of rescue workers

Rescuers will require refreshment. The Police will activate the WRVS (Women's Royal Voluntary Service) or the Salvation Army as part of their Major Incident Plan, so that mobile canteen facilities are quickly available.

Law and order

The scene of a major incident is a scene of crime. Evidence must be protected for use in later criminal proceedings.

In the case of a large scale evacuation of the public, empty properties present soft targets for opportunist thieves and looters. The Police are responsible for the protection of property.

The media

The Police will provide a Press Liaison Officer and set up a Media Liaison Point beyond the outer cordon. Further details of how to deal with the media are given in Chapter 10.

POLICE AID TO THE HEALTH SERVICES

The Police can assist the Health Services at the scene of a major incident as shown in Box 6.4.

Box 6.4. Police aid to the Medical Services

- Assist with team transport either directly or by providing an escort
- Provide communications on the command net at the scene
- Maintain clear transport routes to ensure the uninhibited movement of ambulances
- Provide escorts for individual casualties to hospital
- Collate information on the whereabouts of the injured and their condition
- Provide a Survivor Reception Centre
- Supervise the provision of food and drink for the rescuers
- Provide conference facilities for incident officer briefings or media statements
- Provide a helicopter(s) for aerial assessment of the scene or the transport of individual casualties

---

Summary

- The Police are in overall control at the scene
- In the presence of fire or chemical hazard the Senior Fire Officer will assume control of the Bronze (operational) area
- The Casualty Bureau will collate all information about the survivors, injured, and dead
- The Police can provide considerable assistance to the Health Services at the scene of a major incident

CHAPTER 7

The Fire Service

After reading this chapter you should be able to answer the following questions:

- What is the organisation and rank structure of the Fire Service?
- What is the meant by a "predetermined attendance"?
- What is the role of the Fire Service at a major incident?
- How can the Fire Service assist the Health Services at a major incident?

ORGANISATION

The divisional organisation of the operational aspects of the Fire Service is shown in Figure 7.1, and the organisation of a fire station is shown in Figure 7.2.

A typical division may have eight or nine fire stations, with approximately 380 personnel.

RANK STRUCTURE

The rank structure of the British Fire Service is shown in Figure 7.3.

The epaulette and helmet markings of the Fire Service are shown in Figure 7.4.

PREDETERMINED ATTENDANCE

The Fire Service has a statutory obligation under the Fire Services' Act to ensure that all calls to fires are attended by pumping appliances within a specified time. The time taken to respond and the number of vehicles initially dispatched match the perceived risk and are termed the "predetermined attendance" (PDA).

For example, a call to a fire in a rural area requires only one appliance to attend within 20 minutes, whereas a call to a city centre fire will require three appliances, two of which must arrive within five minutes and the third within eight minutes. For a motorway incident it is recommended that two pumping appliances are mobilised simultaneously, which will approach the incident from opposite carriageways, to ensure that the incident is covered; additionally, an emergency tender or light rescue vehicle may be dispatched when casualties are trapped.

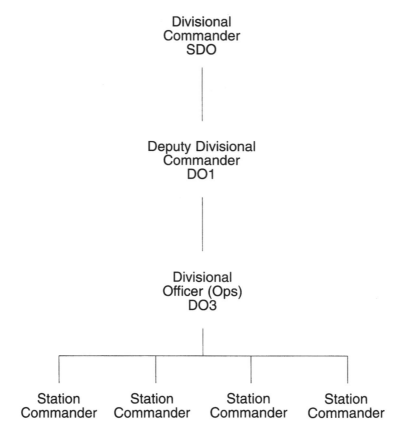

Figure 7.1.   Divisional organisation of the Fire Service

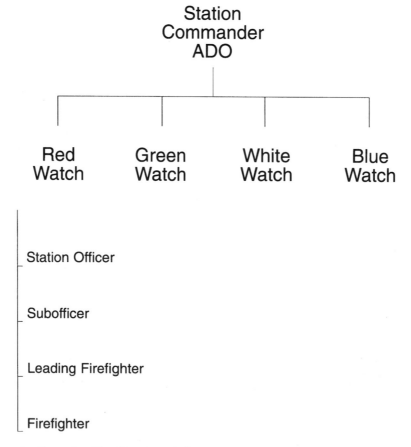

Figure 7.2.   Organisation of a Fire Service station

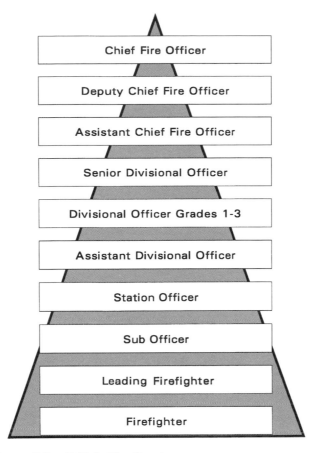

Figure 7.3. Rank structure of the British Fire Service

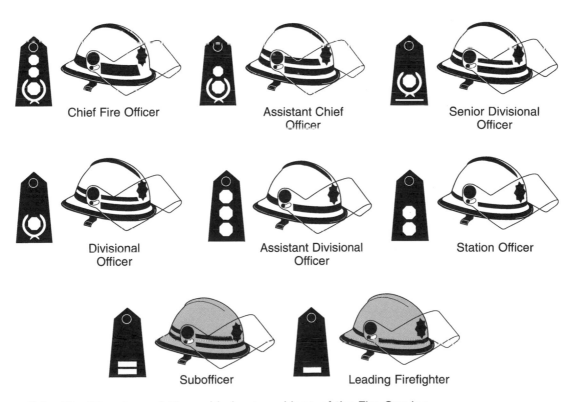

Figure 7.4. Traditional epaulette and helmet markings of the Fire Service

> **A Senior Fire Service Officer has a white helmet. The number and width of the bands denote rank**

The PDA will also determine the rank of the initial officer to be mobilised. As an example, it is suggested that an officer of rank of Assistant Divisional Officer or above is sent to the scene if people are known to be trapped or dangerous substances are involved.

In each area there will be a number of high risk areas such as an airport or petrochemical works. These are potential sites for major incidents and the initial response to a call from such an area will be above the standard requirement.

The importance of the predetermined attendance is that it ensures that the initial response of the Fire Service, *before* a major incident is declared, involves multiple vehicles and multiple personnel (including a senior officer); this corresponds with perceived risk on receipt of the first 999 call. This is unlike the Police or Ambulance Service whose initial response will often only be a single vehicle.

> **The predetermined attendance ensures an adequate initial response and the presence of an appropriately senior officer at all incidents**

Major incident predetermined attendance

Box 7.1 shows the predetermined attendance for a major incident in Greater Manchester County. Other counties may differ slightly.

Box 7.1. Major incident predetermined attendance	
Pumping appliances	10
Emergency salvage tenders	2
Foam tender	1
Control unit	1

In addition to the resources listed in Box 7.1 five pumping appliances are mobilised to the nearest fire station, and this station is then used as a rendezvous point for further resources. As appliances are sent forward from the rendezvous point to the incident, more are requested to the rendezvous point to maintain a pool of five pumping appliances.

Extraordinary mobilising scheme

In many cases a simple, compensated, major incident can be dealt with by calling upon resources within the one county. It is recognised, however, that there may be a need to call upon resources from surrounding areas.

The object of this extraordinary mobilising scheme is to provide an additional 50 pumping appliances to any incident within the area of the participating authorities. As an example, in the north-west region of England, the county Fire Services have agreed to provide the following maximum number of pumping appliances, subject to their availability at the time:

Greater Manchester	20
Lancashire	15
Merseyside	15
Cheshire	10
Clwyd	5
Cumbria	5
Gwynedd	5

This scheme will be implemented when any participating authority receives a request from the fire ground for more appliances than can be provided under normal local mobilisation procedures.

Fire Service special appliances

The Fire Service has a number of special appliances that are operationally available and which may form part of the predetermined attendance to a specific incident. These appliances are listed below.

Control unit
This unit has a specialist support crew and attends all major incidents. It provides the Senior Fire Officer at the scene with pre-prepared plans for dealing with anticipated incidents within the Brigade area, together with communications (radio, facsimile, and telephone), maps, and incident conference facilities. This appliance may also act as the information centre for press enquiries, and will provide the essential link between the incident site and the Central Brigade Control.

Emergency salvage tender
This vehicle carries sealed major incident kits. It also carries equipment for the following:

- Hazardous substance and radiation related incidents, for example, gas tight, one piece suit, equipment for monitoring radiation contamination, equipment for decontamination
- Floods and protection of buildings from water damage during firefighting, for example, a variety of pumps.

Aerial appliance
This may be a turntable ladder or hydraulic platform (or a combination of these). They can deliver up to 3300 litres of water per minute (a standard pumping appliance will only carry about 1800 litres of water).

Foam tender and high expansion (HI-EX) foam unit
These two appliances provide the means necessary to deal with flammable liquid fires. The HI-EX foam generators can also be used for smoke extraction.

Breathing apparatus tender
This appliance provides a complete breathing appliance (BA) servicing facility and will become the breathing apparatus main control in large or protracted BA incidents.

Light rescue vehicle (LRV) and inshore rescue boat

The LRV is mobilised to motorway incidents. It provides a fourwheel drive capability and carries a scaled down version of the equipment on the emergency salvage tender.

The inshore rescue boat is equipped for casualty rescue from inland waterways.

Hose laying vehicle

This carries large diameter hose and is deployed when there are inadequate supplies of water available near to the scene of the fire.

ROLE OF THE FIRE SERVICE AT A MAJOR INCIDENT

The officer in charge of the first appliance to arrive at the incident will make an assessment of the scene and radio an "assistance message" to Fire Service Control. This message will include the term "major incident," and the information contained in Table 7.1.

Table 7.1. Initial information to be passed from the scene of a major incident

E	Exact location	Grid reference
T	Type of incident	Rail, chemical, road
H	Hazards	Current and potential
A	Access	From which direction to approach
N	Number of casualties	And their severity/type
E	Emergency services	Present and required

This officer must then formulate a plan and implement this by clear instructions to his subordinates. He must monitor the situation to ensure that these instructions are carried out fully and effectively, and that any developments in the situation are also controlled. The initial responsibilities of the Fire Service are given in Box 7.2.

Box 7.2. Fire Service initial responsibilities

Establishment of a forward control
Saving of life
Prevention of escalation of the incident
Fighting of fires
Elimination of hazards
Rescuing entrapped casualties
Clearing routes in and out of the wreckage
Liaison with the other emergency services
Provision of specialist equipment (lighting, lifting, tentage)
Freeing the dead

Two problems may beset the Fire Service early in the major incident. These are *access* and a continuing *supply of water*. Access may be difficult if the incident occurs away from a main road (such as on a railway line or in a tunnel). The water carried by a pumping appliance can be rapidly consumed in a severe fire. It is then necessary to take water from hydrants, streams, rivers, ponds, and any other sources that are available locally.

The Fire Service is a disciplined service and trains its firefighters to react to an order by performing a "drill" (that is, a series of actions the nature of which are predetermined). This helps to maintain the speed and efficiency of the team in the most difficult of circumstances. Firefighters are trained to respond to orders and, consequently, may respond poorly to medical personnel who only make weak suggestions. If you need the Fire Service to do something for you, ask for it firmly and specifically—it will then be done.

Section 30 of the Fire Services' Act states that the Senior Fire Officer present has sole charge of operations relating to fire. In practice this can be extended to control of operations in the immediate area of the incident where any hazard exists (for example, chemical spillage, building collapse). It is the Fire Service, therefore, that are often in charge at the Bronze (operational) level, although the Police retain overall control of the scene. Good liaison with other emergency services is imperative, and there should be no confusion as to where responsibilities lie.

The fire officer in charge must be ready to brief a more senior officer, including an appraisal of how the situation is likely to develop, and formally to hand over command.

Duties of the Senior Fire Officer

When a major incident is declared a Senior Divisional Officer or Assistant Chief Officer is required to take command of the Fire Service resources at the scene. The command responsibilities of the officer are shown in Box 7.3.

Box 7.3. Command of Fire Service resources

- Assume command of all Fire Service resources, taking charge of all operations concerned with firefighting, saving life from fire, and rescue of trapped people
- Establish a command post in the Control Unit near to the Police and Ambulance Control Units
- Nominate officers to take charge of various sections of the incident, and nominate safety officers
- Provide special equipment such as pumps, rescue equipment, emergency lighting, and any resources needed from the Local Authority. *Note*: if helicopters or military assistance are needed for Fire Service purposes these are requested at Chief Officer level
- Where fire is not involved, deploy personnel and equipment in liaison with the Senior Police Officer present, and generally assist other services
- Provide or obtain specialist assistance where hazardous substances are involved (see Part VII, Appendix A)

The Senior Fire Officer present is responsible for identifying when his crews should be relieved. Under normal conditions this will be after four hours of work at an incident, but can be reduced to three hours during the night and in extreme conditions (for example, a particularly hot period in breathing apparatus; wet uniform; fatal incidents; or injury involving a firefighter). The senior officer at the scene will dictate the number of appliances and personnel required for relief, but their acquisition is the responsibility of Brigade Control.

FIRE SERVICE AID TO THE HEALTH SERVICES

The Fire Service can assist the Health Services at the scene of a major incident in the ways shown in Box 7.4.

The Fire Service is highly disciplined, highly motivated, and resourceful. It can provide considerable assistance to the Health Services, particularly when dealing with trapped casualties. Clear instructions should be given by the doctor or paramedic to firefighters involved in the release of a casualty.

Box 7.4. Fire Service aid to medical services

- Provide a safe area to work—by removing fire, chemical, electrical, or other hazards, and by clearing routes into and out of the immediate scene
- Provide an improved area to work—with lighting, shelter from a tarpaulin, and improved access to the trapped patient
- Provide skills and equipment to extricate entrapped casualties
- Provide personnel to assist medical procedures (thereby releasing medical staff)—such as manual stabilisation of the cervical spine, supporting fractured limbs, squeezing infusion bags
- Provide personnel to lift and carry casualties from the incident to the Casualty Clearing Station
- Provide first aid when medical resources are limited
- Assist in applying triage labels under the supervision of a doctor, nurse, or paramedic when medical resources are very limited

**Ask the advice of the Fire Service when dealing with a trapped casualty.
Give clear instructions during the extrication**

Summary
- The Senior Fire Officer is the one with the white helmet who has the greatest number and the thickest black bands
- The predetermined attendance ensures an adequate initial response and the presence of an appropriately senior officer at all incidents
- In the presence of fire or other immediate hazard the Senior Fire Officer will assume command in the Bronze (operational) area
- The Fire Service can provide enormous assistance to the Health Services at the scene of a major incident

CHAPTER

8

Support services

After reading this chapter you should be able to answer these questions:

- What support services are available?
- How can these agencies assist the Health Services at the scene of a major incident?

DEFINITION

In this text the support services are those agencies requested to provide assistance at the scene of a major incident which are not part of the Police, Fire Service, Ambulance Service, and hospital Medical Services. They include the following:

- Her Majesty's Coastguard
- The Voluntary Ambulance Services
- Other voluntary societies (Salvation Army; WRVS)
- The radio amateurs network (RAYNET)
- The military
- Local Authority.

SPECIFIC SERVICES

HM Coastguard

The coastguard will have a principal role in coordinating the rescue of casualties from an offshore incident, which they control from a *Maritime Rescue Coordination Centre*. Once on land the organisational structure for the management of a major incident will be identical.

The Voluntary Ambulance Services

The Voluntary Ambulance Services (VAS) are composed of the following:

- British Red Cross
- St John Ambulance Service
- St Andrew Ambulance Service (Scotland).

These societies may be mobilised as part of the Ambulance Service major incident plan, or by the Police following a request from the Ambulance Incident Officer. The aid offered by these societies is listed in Box 8.1.

Box 8.1.   Aid offered by the Voluntary Ambulance Services

Fully equipped ambulances to transport seriously injured to hospital
Staff to look after medical aid posts for minor injured
Staff to look after first aid post in Survivor Reception Centre and rest centres
Transport of minor injured to hospital
Stretcher bearing duties on the scene
Assistance with transporting the dead

Additionally, members may be deployed to the receiving hospitals where they can function as auxiliaries, or they may act as messengers ("runners") on the scene.

Other voluntary societies

These include the following:

● The Salvation Army
● The Women's Royal Voluntary Service (WRVS).

The Salvation Army and WRVS provide practical support such as "tea and sympathy," and in the context of a major incident this support for the emergency services at the scene should not be undervalued. Staff work more efficiently in an uncomfortable environment when they are rested periodically and have access to food and drink. These periods of rest may also be the first opportunity for the rescuers to talk to each other about their experiences and to begin the long, and sometimes painful, debriefing process—this will be facilitated by the relaxed and supportive atmosphere these organisations generate.

Radio amateurs network

The radio amateurs network (RAYNET) may provide staff and equipment to supplement the communications system at the scene. This has been utilised in major incidents to great effect (notably at Lockerbie) to provide a communications link between search teams. If used by the Health Services such a system must be supervised to ensure that all important messages are fed through the Ambulance Service Emergency Control Vehicle.

The military

The Armed Services are a source of large numbers of organised, trained, and disciplined personnel. Their use may depend upon the geographical location of the incident, the time scale, and the ability to be released from military commitments.

In addition to this simple manpower resource the Armed Services have skills that are useful especially when the incident is compound (see Chapter 1)—such as the building of temporary bridges, the preparation of aircraft landing sites, and the provision of field kitchens, shelter, clean water, and hygiene. The military medical services will be able to erect field hospitals in such circumstances.

Specialist parts of the military can be of specific assistance to the civil community. Royal Air Force and Royal Navy search and rescue helicopters are used for both offshore and mountain rescue. In terrorist incidents Army bomb disposal teams will be required to assist the Police in identifying and making safe any *secondary devices* (a second bomb in the same vicinity often specifically intended to injure the emergency services). Where there is a special risk, such as that posed by a nuclear installation, the Armed Services can provide expertise in planning and response that would not be available from a civilian source.

In areas where a permanent military establishment exists it is common for the military to be involved in local major incident planning and to have a predetermined role in the event of an incident. This may be to provide fire, salvage, or rescue resources, or in the vicinity of a military hospital to provide a medical team.

A request for provision of military aid to the scene is directed through the Police Incident Officer. Authorisation may already exist as part of an agreed planned response to an anticipated incident. If it does not it will have to be sought for the first time on the day. Final authority may be given locally but may have to involve the Ministry of Defence or Central Government.

Local Authority

In the acute phase of the major incident response the Local Authority can provide assistance to the emergency services and support to the community; in the longer term the Local Authority will have a primary role in the recovery of the community.

Support to the emergency services

Initially the response will be to provide machinery and plant to assist in the rescue operation: earth moving equipment may be needed to clear routes; steps can be laid on embankments; additional lighting can be provided. Public transport can be used for casualty evacuation. Shelter will be made available for rest centres with provision for food and drinks; those who require temporary accommodation will be housed.

Long term recovery

Over weeks or months the Local Authority Social Services will continue to care for those survivors who are vulnerable to post-traumatic stress disorder (see Part VII, Appendix B).

Cleansing, environmental health, housing, public works, and building departments may all be involved in the reconstruction of the community.

Summary
- Support services are available to complement the regular Police, Fire Service, Ambulance Service, and medical response to a major incident
- The Ambulance Incident Officer can request the help of the Voluntary Ambulance Services
- Local Authority services are essential both to the initial response and to the longer term reconstruction of communities

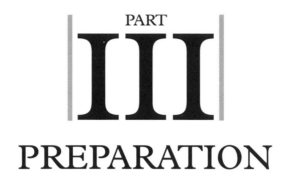

PART

III

PREPARATION

CHAPTER

9

Personal equipment

After reading this chapter you should be able to answer the following questions:

- What are the minimum safe clothing requirements for pre-hospital care?
- What additional items of clothing and personal equipment are desirable to improve comfort and efficiency?

MINIMUM CLOTHING

The following are the most important considerations for pre-hospital care clothing:

- Personal safety
- Function and durability
- Comfort.

Doctors in white coats and flip-flops or nurses in uniform are a liability both to themselves and to others at the scene of a major incident. Individuals who are inappropriately dressed should be refused entry to the scene—this is the responsibility of the Ambulance Safety Officer and the Medical Incident Officer. In spite of this advice, such individuals have still been seen at recent incidents.

> **Individuals who are inappropriately dressed or equipped will be denied access by the Ambulance Safety Officer**

Personal safety for the rescuers must be the first priority at the scene. To achieve this, each rescuer must be visible and protected against the probable hazards, including the elements, glass, sharp metal, fire, and blood. Box 9.1 lists the areas of the body that must be protected and Box 9.2 lists the minimum clothing requirements.

59

Box 9.1. Body areas that must be protected

Vulnerable areas
- Head
- Face/eyes
- Ears
- Body
- Hands
- Feet

Box 9.2. Minimum clothing requirements

Hard hat, with visor or additional goggles
Ear defenders
Warm underclothing
Fire retardant suit
High visibility jacket, marked appropriately
Heavy duty gloves
Latex gloves
Oil and acid resistant boots

In cold weather, *warm underclothing* is important. A *fire retardant suit* should be worn on top of this. Some suits have knee and elbow pads which are useful when working on the floor. If suits are not on personal issue, potential rescuers must make sure that they know the size that fits. A *high visibility reflective jacket* should be worn over this suit: the conventional colours for the medical services are a jacket with green yoke and yellow lower half. The jacket should be clearly labelled on the front and back (the colour of lettering will be green on white). The Incident Officers will also wear a green and white chequered tabard labelled front and rear.

A *hard hat* is mandatory. Hats have the tendency to fall off and a helmet with a secure chin strap is recommended. The colour of helmet will be green with white lettering for doctors and nurses, and white with green lettering for the Ambulance Service. The helmet should be of high specification (that is, Kevlar composite). A torch can be mounted on the helmet which will allow both hands to remain free. The eyes must be protected by a *visor* or Perspex *goggles*. Strong footwear is needed: *boots* should be oil and acid resistant. Wellington boots are commonly stocked by hospitals for pre-hospital use, but are barely adequate for any climbing around the scene. Both a *heavy duty pair of gloves* (to protect against glass and sharp metal) and a pair of *latex gloves* (to protect against blood) are needed. The ears are protected (from the loud background noise of the Fire Service generators and cutting equipment) by *ear defenders*.

Standardisation of clothing is important to prevent confusion between emergency service personnel, and to aid identification from a distance.

ADDITIONAL ITEMS

Additional items of personal equipment that may be carried are listed below:

- *Identification*
  This is essential because rescuers may not be allowed on the scene if they arrive independently and are unable to prove their identity.

- *Notebook*
- *Aide memoire and action cards*
  As a minimum each rescuer should have an action card listing priorities at the scene. Little effort is required to construct a personal *aide memoire*, which can be waterproofed (for example, by placing the pages inside a pocket sized photograph album).
- *Camera*
  It is not a legal requirement to obtain consent before photography, but any photograph taken can later be demanded for legal evidence. A Polaroid photograph can accompany a patient if this will help in the further management (it may assist the hospital staff in appreciating the mechanism and severity of an injury).
- *Torch*
  A helmet torch is recommended.
- *Whistle*
- *Money*
  This can help with communications and with getting home if stranded.

These additional items, together with personal refreshments and combination of items (scissors; penknife; basic treatment kit—airway, dressing, pocket mask) can be conveniently carried in pouches on a belt.

Summary
- All Health Service staff must adhere to minimum clothing requirements
- Any who are incorrectly dressed will be refused entry to the scene by the Ambulance Safety Officer or Medical Incident Officer
- Clothing should conform to national standards to aid recognition and prevent confusion

CHAPTER

10

Medical equipment

After reading this chapter you should be able to answer the following questions:

- Why is extra medical equipment necessary?
- What equipment is required for first aid?
- What equipment is required for advanced life support?
- How should a Mobile Medical Team's equipment be packed?
- How is extra medical equipment delivered to the scene?

INTRODUCTION

As with all aspects of major incident care, the provision of medical equipment requires forward planning. Equipment requirements are different from normal pre-hospital care for two main reasons. First, the *number* of casualties will be much larger than under normal circumstances. Second, the *time* elapsed before casualties arrive at hospital, and therefore the time spent on scene providing treatment, may be greatly increased—not only as a result of entrapment, but also because of the casualty numbers exceeding the transport capacity for evacuation. Together these factors mean that the attending ambulances have insufficient supplies to treat all the casualties. Extra provision must be made for this necessary equipment, and this provision will be met by both the Ambulance Service and the Mobile Medical Teams.

> **Extra equipment must be provided both by the Ambulance Service and by the Mobile Medical Teams**

The Mobile Medical Team must supply any equipment necessary for advanced procedures not normally performed by paramedics.

FIRST AID

The type of equipment used for first aid is similar to that used by the Ambulance Service on a day to day basis. The principal difference in a major incident is the quantity that will be required. As triage and the treatment of immediately life threatening

63

conditions (those threatening the ABCs—airway, breathing, circulation) are the initial actions of the "first aider," the equipment should reflect this.

Triage labels are an essential part of the first aid pack. The most important equipment will be for airway control and the arrest of exsanguinating external haemorrhage—thus a supply of oral and nasopharyngeal airways and absorbent gauze pressure dressings is paramount.

> **Initially simple equipment for ABC management is all that is needed**

Triage labels

Triage labels should be easily and securely attached to patients, must be marked and colour coded for priority, and must be made of an appropriate material (see Chapter 16). They should also be weather resistant but still allow writing with a variety of markers. As triage is a dynamic process it must be possible to recategorise the patients rapidly, without having to rewrite all the notes.

> **Triage labels are an essential part of the first aid pack**

For all these reasons cruciform triage labels are the best available, and an adequate supply must be included in all medical equipment packs.

ADVANCED LIFE SUPPORT

Advanced life support will be administered at the Casualty Clearing Station. The equipment needs of such an area are familiar to those who work in emergency medicine, because the main requirement is for large amounts of equipment for stabilisation of ABCs. There are a number of ways of arranging the supply and resupply of this area.

One way is to arrange items in patient sets, that is, one complete set of equipment for control of ABC per patient. In this scheme a box stays by each patient and equipment is consequently close at hand if required urgently. Although this leads to a degree of overprovision, it avoids the confusion that can arise when searching for equipment from a central storage area. Resupply is simple because the set of equipment can be returned to the equipment vehicle for replenishment once the casualty leaves the scene.

An alternative scheme is to keep non-disposable items (such as self inflating bags and laryngoscopes) in a central area, and issue boxes of disposable items (such as dressings, airways, intravenous cannulas, and fluids) either in single or multi-patient packs. This avoids the problem of supplying expensive items to each individual casualty area. Resupply of the boxes of disposable items is from a central store.

Mobile Medical Team equipment

Mobile Medical Teams must be appropriately equipped to the standards described above and should have access to those items listed in Box 10.1. Their equipment must be coordinated with the Ambulance Service but should not merely duplicate it, because they can carry out more procedures and administer more drugs than ambulance paramedics.

Box 10.1. Examples of equipment carried by Mobile Medical Teams

Advanced airway
  Difficult intubation
  Cricothyroidotomy

Advanced breathing
  Chest drains
  Chest drainage bags

Advanced circulation
  High flow cannulas
  Pressure infusors

Advanced drugs
  Local and regional anaesthesia
  Opiate analgesia
  General anaesthesia

Advanced trauma
  Traction splints

Surgical equipment
  Cut down equipment
  Amputation

Mobile Medical Team equipment should be compatible with Ambulance Service equipment. It should supplement rather than duplicate, and must reflect the extended skills of the team

---

Mobile Medical Teams should therefore either carry equipment for advanced procedures to the scene, or make prior arrangements for it to be stored in Ambulance Service equipment vehicles. The Mobile Medical Team should be equipped to undertake any procedures that may be required in the first hour of onsite care. Of particular importance is the need to carry both sufficient analgesics for parenteral administration and some local anaesthetic agents for use in regional blocks. It is important that, if the contents of the Mobile Medical Teams' bags are significantly different to those in the standard issue bags, the two can be readily distinguished. This can be achieved either by appropriate written marking, or by using a different colour of bag.

Mobile Medical Team equipment should be clearly identifiable

Immediate care doctors

In some areas the responsibility for medical care at major incidents may rest with immediate care doctors. They usually only carry equipment for the treatment of relatively small numbers of casualties. Arrangements therefore need to be made with local hospitals or with the Ambulance Service to supply equipment that would otherwise be brought by the hospital based Mobile Medical Team.

RESUPPLY FROM HOSPITAL

Occasionally an unexpected procedure will be required. In this circumstance the Medical Incident Officer (MIO) should have a contact point at the local hospital to arrange the supply of this equipment or drug. A prearranged procedure should be in place to guarantee the timely delivery of the correct item to the correct person (MIO).

Blood

The MIO should also ensure that the blood transfusion service is present at the site if required. They can not only provide blood and crossmatching facilities, but also equipment for blood and fluid administration in large quantities.

Standardisation

Each person works best with equipment sets with which he is familiar. However, standardisation of equipment sets is better than personalisation because a number of different organisations will often share equipment in a major incident.

> **Standardisation of equipment allows interchangeability between rescuers, and easy resupply**

The best arrangement is to have a universally agreed type of equipment bag organised in a standard manner. All personnel can use this and, when it runs short of supplies, it can simply be replaced by a full bag.

A bag and box system is shown in Boxes 10.2 and 10.3.

National standardisation

Ideally major incident equipment sets should be standardised nationally, as is the case in France. If this were the case in the United Kingdom then all rescuers could be made familiar with the contents and layout during training. As it is, at best this can currently only be achieved at a local level.

CONTAINERS

Various types of container can be considered to carry the equipment—but a key factor in choosing the design must be its ease of use in difficult circumstances. The container should be designed to be comfortable to carry over a long distance or difficult terrain, and the contents should be visible, accessible, and secure even if held upside down.

Containers should be easy to carry and keep equipment visible, accessible, and secure

For these reasons rucksacks that have multiple pockets with clear fronts are popular. Many teams use plastic boxes which may or may not have been specifically designed for the task. Just as with rucksacks these must provide sufficient storage for the equipment supplied, and must allow easy access along with security for the contents.

All Mobile Medical Team equipment should be checked regularly both for completeness and to ensure that all items are serviceable and in date.

Regular checking by the staff who will use the equipment has a useful training function in that it encourages familiarity with both the equipment itself and the way in which it is stored.

EQUIPMENT VEHICLES

Most Ambulance Services have one or more mobile equipment units ("emergency support units") which can be rapidly deployed to the scene of a major incident. The exact number and distribution of these vary, but most Ambulance Services would aim to have the equipment unit to the scene within 20 minutes.

Some services use trailer units whereas others use specifically designed vehicles; local conditions will determine which is most appropriate. Whatever the design, it is important that the vehicle is clearly marked as the Central Equipment Supply. Some services have put combined control and equipment units into service; this is less than ideal because a conflict of interest in deployment can occur.

The broad nature of the equipment likely to be found on a particular vehicle is discussed above. The exact amount will be determined according to both the incidents expected to occur within the operational area and the number of vehicles deployed. As a general rule major incident equipment vehicles carry enough equipment to treat 60 casualties. If the incident involves more casualties than this then the equipment vehicle from the neighbouring area should also be summoned. In the case of prolonged incidents, arrangements must be in place for the Regional Health Care supplies unit to be opened so that the equipment vehicles can be replenished.

Equipment Officer

If there is more than one equipment vehicle at the scene it is important that an ambulance officer is designated as the Ambulance Equipment Officer. Mobile Medical Teams may leave their resupply and surplus specialist equipment with this officer and, if sufficient teams are deployed, may wish to appoint a Medical Equipment Officer to coordinate the central control of their equipment.

The Equipment Officer must ensure that issuing of stores is done rationally and in a controlled fashion. Certain items (such as the Ambulance Incident Officer's tabard) must be strictly controlled if a scene is to be effectively managed. Other items (such as drugs) should be issued only to appropriately qualified and trained staff. If more than one equipment vehicle is in attendance it is essential that each vehicle is depleted in turn and then sent for restocking.

Box 10.2. Medical first response rucksack

(Non-disposables—two major casualties' disposables)

INTRAVENOUS 1
Gelofusine 500 ml × 2
Physiological (normal) saline 500 ml × 2
Blood giving sets × 4

AIRWAY 1

Bandage one inch	Lignocaine jelly
Catheter mount	Magill forceps
Chest drain bags (two)	Minitrach II Set
Endotracheal tubes 7, 8 (two), 9	Portable suction device
Guedel airways 2, 3, 4	Broad tape
Introducer (ETT)	Suction catheters—Yankauer/Soft Tipped
Laryngoscope	Syringe (20 ml)
Self inflating bag	

Chest drains (two)—cervical collars

AIRWAY 2

Laerdal pocket mask

Nasopharyngeal
airways 6, 7, 8

Oxygen masks (high
concn) × 2

INTRAVENOUS 2

Blood sample kits		Needles 21 g × 8
Urea and electroytes		Syringes 20 ml × 4
Full blood count	} kits	3 way taps × 2
Crossmatched blood		Tourniquet
Elastoplast 7·5		Tape 2·5 cm
Gauze squares		Cannulas 16 g × 4
Gloves 4 pairs		Cannulas 18 g × 2
ID bands × 2		

Sharps pad underneath

DRUGS 1—BLACK
Ketamine
Lignocaine
Naloxone

DRUGS 2—YELLOW
Kept in CD Safe

Morphine
Prochlorperazine
Phone card/10p coins

INSTRUMENTS

Clips × 3
Mosquitos × 3
Needle holder
Pen torch
Pens
Scalpel 23 × 4
Scissors—large
Scissors—small
Silk W791 × 4
Tooth forceps

DRESSINGS

Ambulance
dressings
× 4

FRONT POUCH
MIO tabard
Cruciform triage cards × 20
Forms on clipboard
Equipment used (5)
Incident report (5)

Maps
Local A–Z
Predicted sites
Motorway access

Aide memoires
Phone numbers
Equipment
Triage

Action cards
MIO
FMIO
Casualty clearing
Station Officer
Secondary Triage
Officer

Box 10.3. Medical major incident box loading list

MAJOR INCIDENT BOX
(Four major casualties—disposables)

Contents list inside lid
Sharp pad on flap

Top compartment

10 ml syringe × 2 Tape 2.5 cm	23 scalpels × 4 10 ml syringe × 2	Laryngoscope bulb Pens × 4 Marking pen Pen torch	Scissors Batteries × 4 Tourniquet Controlled analgesic drugs	18 g Venflon × 4 16 g Venflon × 5	18 g Venflon × 1 16 g Venflon × 5	21 g needles × 10 ——— Sterets

Middle shelf

Endotracheal tubes
9 × 1
8 × 2
7 × 1

Nasopharyngeal airways
8 × 1
7 × 2
6 × 1

Guedel airways
4 × 2
3 × 2
2 × 2

Gauze squares × 10
20 ml syringes × 2
Lignocaine gel
Minitrach II Set

Oxygen masks (high flow) × 4

Bottom compartment

Physiological (normal) saline 500 ml × 4

Gelofusine 500 ml × 4

Giving sets × 4

Chest drain bags × 2

Crossmatch sets × 4

Gloves × 10

Chest drains × 2

Mobile Medical Team equipment must be checked and serviced regularly

An Equipment Officer should be nominated to ensure the rational use of stores

The Equipment Officer's most difficult task is to ensure that equipment is appropriately issued for use in the inner cordon. Often several requests arrive from varying sources for the same equipment for one patient, leading to a waste of resources. On other occasions equipment will get diverted en route and the requesting team will never receive the item. A system needs to be developed to ensure wherever possible that the correct equipment successfully reaches the correct patient.

Summary
- Extra equipment will be necessary to deal with major incidents
- This equipment is required for basic and advanced control of the ABCs and for triage
- The choice of container is important—both rucksacks and boxes have their place
- The Ambulance Service will provide equipment vehicles at the scene, and should also nominate an Equipment Officer to distribute supplies

11

Communications

After reading this chapter you should be able to answer the following questions:

- Why are good communications important?
- What are the methods of communication at a major incident?
- What is the principle of a radio net?

Radio use and voice procedure are discussed in Chapter 20.

INTRODUCTION

Communications are central to the operation of the major incident response—without good communications the emergency services cannot function as a team. Poor communication is recurrently identified as a problem when major incident management is investigated. Some recent comments are shown below.

> *"I was left with the clear impression that opportunities to*
> *pass vital information between the services were missed."*
> Desmond Fennell, OBE, QC
> Investigation into the King's Cross Underground Fire
>
> *"Emergency services shall carry out exercises simulating a*
> *Major Incident on a regular basis to test specifically their communication*
> *systems in the light of the shortcomings identified . . . "*
> Anthony Hidden, QC
> Investigation into the Clapham Junction Railway Accident

The Ambulance Service has overall responsibility for planning, providing, and coordinating Health Service communications at major incidents, although individual hospitals retain the responsibility for ensuring that there are adequate initial communications.

Poor communications can be considered in terms of the following:

- Lack of information
- Lack of confirmation
- Lack of coordination.

> **Good communications are central to the efficient management of a major incident**

COMMUNICATION METHODS

The following methods of communication will be discussed:

- The radio
- The telephone (cellular; land lines)
- Other methods (runner; television and radio broadcasts; hand signals).

The radio

Before you use the radio it is important to know the following:

- To whom you can speak—the radio net
- How to operate the radio—the working parts
- The correct form of speech—radio voice procedure.

The radio net
Everyone who uses the radio has an identifying name or number—this is a "call sign." Everyone who uses a radio tuned to a specified frequency is part of a "radio net." Each emergency service operates on a separate frequency and therefore has its own net. Messages are usually passed from an individual to a central control room, conventionally call sign "zero" or "control." An example of a radio net is shown in Figure 11.1. "Control" can hear everyone and speak to everyone, but individuals may only be able to hear and speak to "control," depending upon the operating system.

Single frequency simplex—All users transmit and receive on the same, single frequency—all can be heard by, and can speak to, each other provided each set is powerful enough.

Two frequency simplex—Users transmit and receive on separate frequencies. Each user can only talk directly to, and can only hear, "control" (unless "control" organises *talk-through*). "Control" can speak to and hear all stations. This is the usual Ambulance Service system.

If a user has a hand held radio as well as a radio in a vehicle, it is traditional for the same call sign to be used whichever radio is being operated at the time.

Radios will either operate on VHF (very high frequency) or UHF (ultra high frequency). VHF radios have a considerably longer range. Standard Ambulance Service radios will be VHF, and a VHF hand set used at the scene could communicate with the Emergency Control Vehicle (ECV), with ambulance control, and directly with the hospital if they have a VHF set installed. UHF radios may be distributed on the scene for use by key personnel, but are unlikely to have a range that will allow communication much beyond the ECV.

The Ambulance Service is responsible for providing radio communications at the site of an incident, from the incident to ambulance control, and at receiving hospitals. These are dealt with as shown in Box 11.1.

72

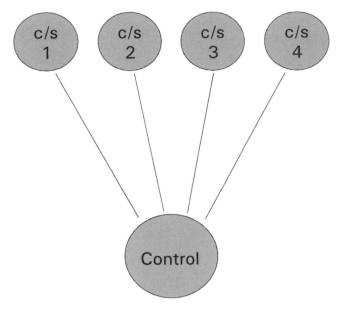

Figure 11.1. A radio net

Only one person can use any radio net at any one time

Box 11.1. Responsibility of Ambulance Service for radio communications

Onsite
The Emergency Control Vehicle will provide the equipment to allow radio communications between:

- Key ambulance and medical staff at the incident
- The incident and the receiving hospitals
- Ambulance vehicles at the scene
- Ambulance control
- The Police and Fire Services

Offsite
Ambulance control will establish and maintain radio communications with:

- The Emergency Control Vehicle at the scene
- Ambulance vehicles travelling to the scene or to hospital
- The receiving hospitals
- The Health Authority
- The Ambulance Services of adjacent Health Authorities

At the hospital
Many accident and emergency departments will have a fixed radio set allowing direct communication with the local Ambulance Service control. In these cases a liaison officer may be dispatched to man the radio at the hospital. Otherwise, a radio set and antenna will be provided by the Ambulance Service

Radio working parts and voice procedure
Chapter 20 contains a detailed description of the radio working parts and how to construct a radio message. Worked examples are given there.

> **Air time is valuable. If you have nothing to say, stay off the air**

Always consider an alternative way to communicate at the scene other than using the radio (see below—runners).

RAYNET

RAYNET is a voluntary organisation of amateur radio enthusiasts who may be called upon to provide supplementary radio communications at the scene of a major incident (see Chapter 8).

The telephone

Cellular telephone

The cellular telephone has a considerable attraction as a communication tool in pre-hospital care. It has the following advantages:

- It allows free conversational speech—radio voice procedure is unnecessary
- It allows direct communication with hospitals
- It has nationwide coverage
- It allows communication with individuals outside the radio net.

There are, however, disadvantages to the use of cellular telephones at a major incident:

- There is no central control of messages
- There are limited cells available which may quickly be occupied.

The absence of central control of messages will mean that important requests are not logged by the Ambulance ECV, and these requests will not be routinely followed up if they fail to materialise. It also leads to a duplication of efforts, counterorders, and a break down in the control of the scene.

The problem of a limited number of cells rapidly being occupied (often by members of the press, who respond almost as quickly as the emergency services) can be overcome by instituting *Access Overload Control* or ACCOLC. At the request of the Police only those cellular telephones that are registered with the Home Office, and which have received the authorised software modification, will continue to function on a number of restricted cells. Other telephones are temporarily disconnected. Clearly there must have been forethought to ensure that an incident officer's telephone is protected in this way.

> **Messages *must* be passed through the Ambulance ECV to maintain control of the scene**

Land lines

In protracted incidents it may be possible to install a number of land line telephones in the field. These emergency telephone services can be requested by the Police from service providers.

Within a hospital the telephone is the principal form of communication. As on the radio, messages should be kept short. Additional telephone points may be necessary within areas designated for major incident administration inside the hospital, although telephones will only be put into use when the plan is activated. Facsimile (fax) points will also be required (a common request of the Police Documentation Team, who will set up a station within the accident and emergency department). The use of a fax can also simplify the transfer of documentation from the site to the hospital.

The hospital switchboard will be rapidly saturated with calls in a major incident. It is the responsibility of the hospital's managers to provide a system that will cope with the increase in demand of calls, and to test this system regularly. It is recommended that dedicated, ex-directory lines are installed to allow Ambulance Control to speak to the accident and emergency department, that these telephones are configured to prevent outgoing calls, and that the line is tested at least once weekly.

Other methods

Runners

In the field the use of runners should always be considered. They are reliable and often faster than trying to make contact over a very busy radio net. It is wise to send hand written messages to avoid "Chinese whispers." The job of runner may not be popular, and it is inappropriate to divert the skills of an ambulanceman or nurse to this task. Members of the voluntary services (St John's, Red Cross, Salvation Army) may be willing to support the emergency services in this role.

Runners are reliable and may be faster than using the radio

The use of runners is also possible within a hospital.

Hand signals

Hand signals can be adopted, but their meaning must have been agreed in advance.

Whistles

A whistle can be used to good effect to attract attention, but close liaison with other services about the meaning of various signals is necessary. As an example, whistle blasts are used by the Fire Service to indicate imminent danger and the need to evacuate the site. Clearly the use of similar signals by other services may cause confusion.

Public announcements

A megaphone may augment scene control and allow brief messages to be passed and collective instructions can be announced over a tannoy (public address system).

Television and radio broadcasts

In certain circumstances the broadcasting media can be used to the advantage of the Health Services. For example, an announcement on local radio can alert off duty staff to attend the hospital immediately. Guidelines do exist, issued by the Home Office, which state the procedure for requesting a BBC broadcast. These guidelines should be incorporated into local Major Incident Plans.

At the scene the Medical Incident Officer should make a request through the Police Incident Officer. At the hospital, if the procedure is unclear, help should be sought from the Regional Health Emergency Planning Officer.

Video

Police or Fire Service videos can be made available at the hospital within a short time and provide a graphic illustration of the problems at the scene, which may assist management decisions. More recently, a direct portable satellite video link with the scene and the emergency service control room has allowed senior officers remote from the scene to determine what additional resources are required.

Satellites

INMARSAT (International Maritime Satellite) and other similar systems allow international portable telephone communications. Many countries subscribe to this system, and the media frequently have access to it. As it does not rely on local infrastructure it is invaluable in large compound incidents.

THE MEDIA

Although the media may occasionally be used to the advantage of major incident management (see above), they are more commonly regarded as a hindrance—and it is not uncommon for a large number of newspaper, radio, and television reporters to attend the scene within a very short time. Firm control is needed, while allowing them adequate access to report the incident.

Media interest in a major incident will be considerable. Initially local newspaper, radio, and television reporters will attend, often arriving at the same time as the emergency services. National and international interest must be anticipated.

At the scene

The media expect to be given the opportunity to report and the privilege of access to photograph, to film, and to talk to key personnel. Uncontrolled they may contaminate the scene of the crime, obstruct the emergency services, and intrude upon the dignity of the injured. Properly respected they can be controlled with regular information, interviews with senior officers, and photograph opportunities. Over-restricted they will resort to unethical tactics to obtain the information they need to meet their production deadlines.

Box 11.2 lists the key areas to address which will produce good media relations while maintaining control.

Box 11.2. Requirements for efficient media handling

Create a media rendezvous point
Restrict access to the scene
Provide a media liaison officer
Consider providing a media centre
Provide regular information updates to coincide with TV/radio bulletins
Do not favour individual representatives
Provide a public relations manager in extended incidents

Media representatives attending the scene should be given a *rendezvous point* which is beyond the outer security cordon. This will allow the Police to maintain control of all personnel entering the scene. *Access* to the scene may be allowed at the discretion of the Police Incident Officer, and passes issued to identify the individuals clearly. It is likely that only a limited number will be given this privilege, for security and safety reasons, and the media should be allowed to choose who their representatives will be (picking, for example, a television crew, a newspaper reporter, a radio crew, and a photographer—known as a "media pool"). It is unwise to favour particular representatives, as others will be encouraged to get the information they need by any means, regardless of whether they have to resort to unreliable eye witnesses or threaten the security of the scene. Parking space for outside broadcast units should be considered, so that access routes are not restricted by large vehicles. Rules for aerial photography must be decided upon early, and emergency flying restrictions imposed if necessary—helicopters are commonly used by the media, but the resultant noise and downdraft may inhibit the work of firefighters, produce hazards to rescuers from flying debris, and destroy or alter forensic evidence.

Police authorities often have a *media liaison officer.* This officer will provide information updates at regular, specified intervals, therefore encouraging the media to wait for this information rather than searching for their own. It is important to avoid injudicious suppositions as to the cause of the incident, which cannot fully be known in the early phases of the rescue operation, and to concentrate on commenting on how the rescue is progressing. This is aided by directing all information through one individual. The media will be offered brief interviews with emergency service incident officers, which can include the Ambulance Medical and Nursing Incident Officer. It is wise to prepare a statement rather than allow a free question interview. Box 11.3 shows the likely flow of questions and Box 11.4 shows a checklist that can be used when preparing for a media interview. The Medical Incident Officer should brief his staff on how to react to an approach by the media—estimates of the number of casualties or dead should not be given unless these have been confirmed.

A *media centre* should be considered in a large or prolonged incident. This may initially be in a command vehicle or a nearby building, and will provide a focal point for continuing media coordination. It should contain communications equipment, an area for briefings, an area to monitor current media broadcasts, and possibly accommodation for the reporters. The Police or Local Authority may be responsible for this centre. This decision should be made at the planning level.

A *public relations manager* can contribute significantly to the smooth handling of the media and running of the media centre. Suitable individuals should also be identified in the planning stages and invited to attend management planning meetings.

At the hospital

The emphasis of media attention will often shift from the scene to the hospital after the initial rescue phase. The hospital management should make provision for a mini-media centre where the media can gather, obtain refreshments, and be briefed at regular

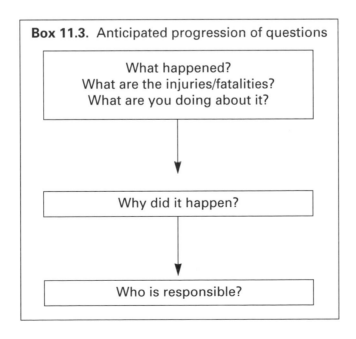

Box 11.3. Anticipated progression of questions

What happened?
What are the injuries/fatalities?
What are you doing about it?

Why did it happen?

Who is responsible?

intervals. Telephones should be available (direct line, avoiding the hospital switchboard). As at the scene, considerate timing of briefings 30–60 minutes before main news bulletins will be appreciated and encourage cooperation.

Senior medical and nursing staff should be aware of the vulnerability of patients, relatives, and staff to intrusive interviews, and should not allow such interviews to interfere with the welfare of patients and the delivery of care. Statements relating to the condition of individual patients or the hospital's response to the major incident are best made by a senior doctor.

Summary
- Good communications are central to the efficient management of a major incident
- All radio users are known by their individual "call sign"
- All radio users on a single frequency constitute a "radio net"
- The uncontrolled use of cellular telephones at the scene may contribute to a loss of scene control
- The media should be dealt with as efficiently as possible

Box 11.4. Checklist for a television interview

Before the interview
Think of your objectives—what are the points you want to get across?
Ask what the first question will be
Ascertain what the "wind up" signal is
Check your appearance

During the interview
Always assume you are on the air
Look straight at the interviewer, not the camera
Avoid jargon, swearing, lying, fidgeting, and losing your cool
Sell yourself: others will be only too ready to criticise
Express sympathy for the injured/dead and their families
Express admiration for the rescue workers and your own staff

After the interview
Stand still until it is clear you are off the air
Distribute copies of any prepared statement

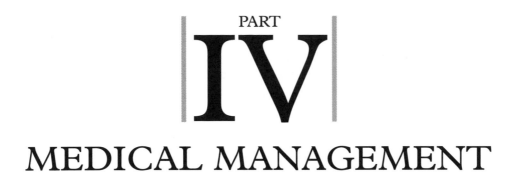

PART

IV

MEDICAL MANAGEMENT

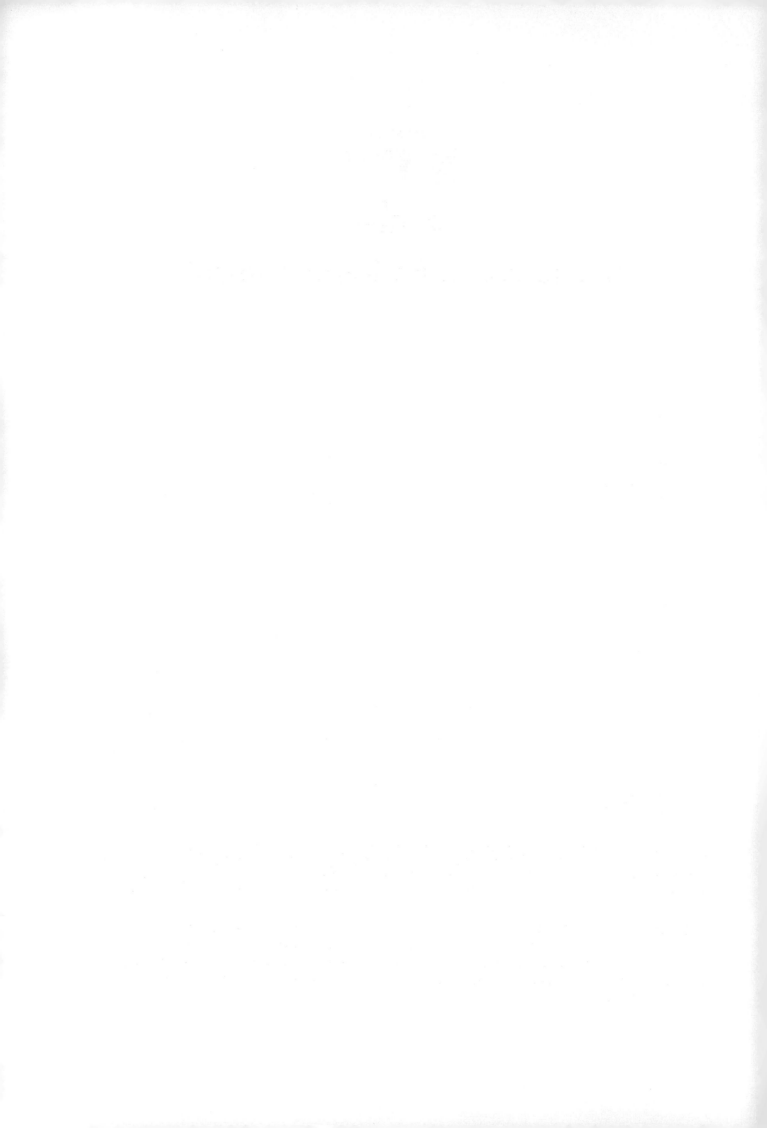

12

Scene command and control

After reading this chapter you should be able to answer these questions:

- Who has overall responsibility at the incident?
- How are the movements of people controlled within the incident?
- What is the chain of command of the emergency services?

OVERALL RESPONSIBILITY

The overall responsibility for the scene of a major incident rests with the Police. The Police should view themselves as facilitators of the other emergency services and ensure their close communication and cooperation.

**Command and control are the cornerstones
of major incident management**

Effective command requires good communication both horizontally (between the incident officers) and vertically (up and down individual service chains of command).

**Good command and control requires good communication
both vertically and horizontally**

In the presence of a fire hazard, the Senior Fire Officer is responsible for controlling the fire. In practical terms the Police will hand the responsibility for controlling any hazard in the immediate area around the incident to the Fire Service. Emergency Health Service personnel entering this hazardous area should ensure that the Senior Fire Officer is aware of their presence.

CONTROL OF MOVEMENT

Movement in and out of the scene of a major incident is controlled by cordoning the area.

Outer cordon

The *outer cordon* will surround the entire incident and will usually encompass an area with a radius of several hundred metres. The outer cordon may consist of Police vehicles blocking streets, traffic cones, tape, or portable metal fencing. It is important that this cordon is a safe distance from any hazard (such as a secondary explosive device) because members of the public and media will gather to observe the incident. Entry and exit through the outer cordon should be strictly controlled through an *Incident Control Point*. Here the Police will keep a timed log of all personnel present working at the incident.

Inner cordon

The *inner cordon*, if marked, will often be surrounded by tape. This is marking the area where the rescue operation is taking place and for Police purposes is the forensic scene of crime. Where a specific hazard exists there may be strict control of personnel entering this area—an inner control point may be set up and all individuals entering the area can be tagged. This record of personnel working in the area will be important if there is a sudden escalation of the incident.

The cordons are illustrated in Figure 12.1.

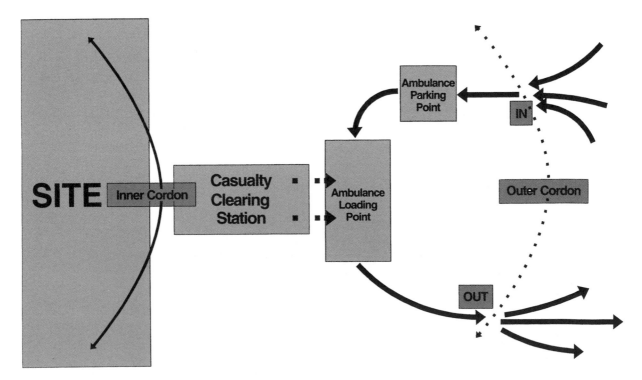

Figure 12.1. The cordons at a major incident

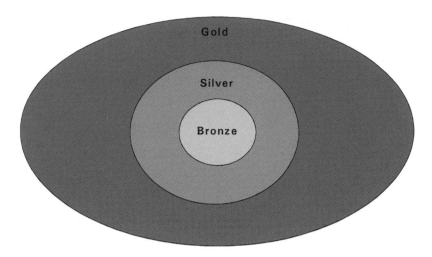

Figure 12.2. The tiers of command

THE TIERS OF COMMAND (Figure 12.2)

The outer cordon marks the area of responsibility of the officers at the scene and therefore is the physical boundary of the Silver (tactical) command. The area of Bronze (operational) command would lie inside the inner cordon; this is somewhat artificial because there may not be a physical boundary, and there may be any number of Bronze areas (for example, individual buildings where people are trapped, or where the wreckage of a train or aircraft is spread over a considerable distance) within the overall scene. When there is more than one Bronze area these are referred to as *sectors*. The Silver commanders may also move around inside the Bronze areas. Gold (strategic) command will be sited some distance from the scene (perhaps Police HQ or the Town Hall) where emergency service chief officers and Local Authority representatives will meet.

THE CHAIN OF COMMAND

Each emergency service must appoint an Incident Officer to command the resources at the scene. In the Police, Fire, and Ambulance Services this role will be handed to more senior officers as they attend. The clinical grade of doctor or nurse is not, however, necessarily related to their suitability to perform the task of Medical or Nursing Incident Officer—individual experience and training are more important (see Chapter 13). The Incident Officers are Silver (tactical) commanders and should interact as shown in Figure 12.3.

The Incident Officers will move around the scene to maintain an overview of how the situation is developing, but will often concentrate their activities close to the line of Incident Control Vehicles inside the outer cordon. It is often the case during major incidents and exercises that barely a word passes between the Incident Officers; the effective management of such a scene demands good communications and these officers *must* arrange to meet at regular intervals.

The Incident Officers are managers and must not be involved directly in the rescue process or the treatment of the injured. It is their job to ensure that there are adequate resources at the scene, and that the resources are maintained through resupply of equipment and replacement of personnel. The organisation of the Silver (tactical) area of command is shown in Figure 12.4.

When there is more than one Bronze (operational) area the Incident Officer may appoint a Forward Incident Officer to manage each sector. Each Bronze (operational)

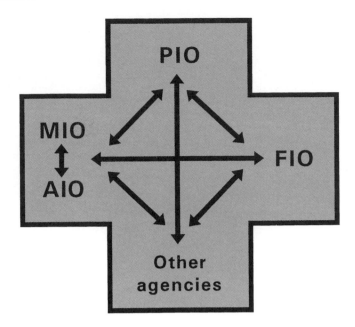

Figure 12.3. The cross of communication: PIO, Police Incident Officer; AIO, Ambulance Incident Officer; FIO, Fire Incident Officer; MIO, Medical Incident Officer

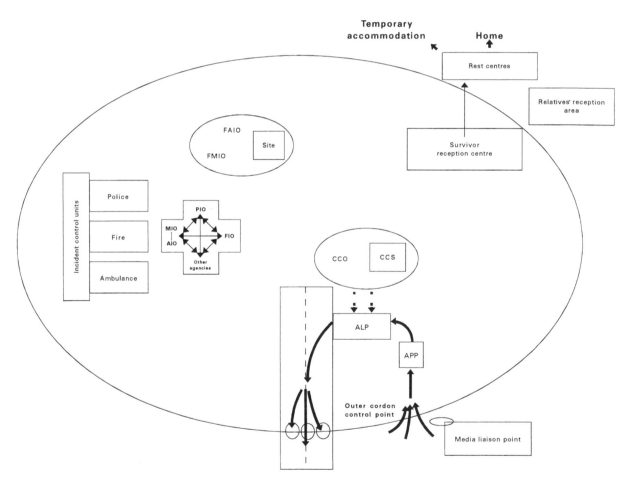

Figure 12.4. The organisation within the Silver (tactical) area of command. MIO, Medical Incident Officer; FMIO, Forward Medical Incident Officer; FIO, Fire Incident Officer; PIO, Police Incident Officer; AIO, Ambulance Incident Officer; FAIO, Forward Ambulance Incident Officer; CCS, Casualty Clearing Station; CCO, Casualty Clearing Officer; ALP, Ambulance Loading Point; APP, Ambulance Parking Point

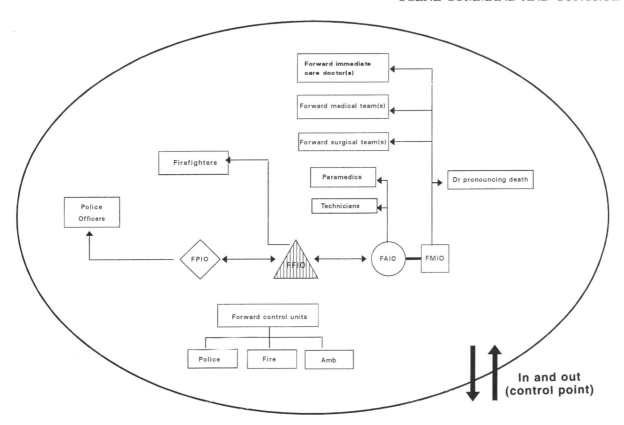

Figure 12.5. The organisation within the Bronze (operational) area of command. FPIO, Forward Police Incident Officer; FFIO, Forward Fire Incident Officer; FAIO, Forward Ambulance Incident Officer; FMIO, Forward Medical Incident Officer; MMT, Mobile Medical Team; MST, Mobile Surgical Team

commander should maintain on overview of his area and report to the Silver commander. The organisation of the Bronze (operational) area of command is shown in Figure 12.5.

Each emergency service has a clearly defined chain of command from the Incident Officer through the Forward Incident Officer to individual personnel on the ground. A request for assistance must be passed through this chain of command to retain control. For example, should a firefighter find a trapped casualty it would seem logical for this firefighter to find the nearest doctor, and take the doctor to the casualty. If this doctor does not request permission for this task, he will be "lost" by the Medical Incident Officer. If this situation is multiplied then all medical resources can be dissipated very rapidly at the scene and control will be compromised.

> **Discipline is required if command and control are to be maintained**

The correct chain of command is for the firefighter to inform his Forward Fire Incident Officer, who will inform the Forward Ambulance Incident Officer (FAIO). The FAIO would send a paramedic to assess the casualty. The paramedic will report back to the FAIO and, if a doctor is required, one will be requested through the Forward Medical Incident Officer by the FAIO.

> **Requests must be passed through the correct chain of command**

Summary

- The Police have overall responsibility at the scene of a major incident
- Good command and control of the incident require good communication both horizontally and vertically
- Entrance and exit through the outer cordon are strictly controlled through an Incident Control Point
- The command structure at the scene is tiered into Silver (tactical) and Bronze (operational) areas. There can be any number of Bronze sectors within the Silver (tactical) area
- Requests for assistance at the scene must pass through the correct chain of command

13

Health Service command and control

After reading this chapter you should be able to answer the following questions:

- Who is in charge of the Health Service response at the scene?
- What are the roles of the Ambulance Incident Officer?
- What are the roles of the Medical Incident Officer?
- What are the roles of a Nursing Incident Officer, and when should one be appointed?
- How is the Health Service response organised on the ground?
- What command tasks are carried out by the Ambulance and Medical Service personnel, who should do these jobs, and where do they occur?

CONTROL OF THE HEALTH SERVICE RESPONSE

As discussed in Chapter 12 the Health Service response is controlled by the Ambulance and Medical Incident Officers. These two officers liaise closely with each other and with the Incident Officers from the Fire and Police Services. Close liaison is essential at this level (Silver control) if the overall response is to be properly coordinated. Both Incident Officers' responsibilities can be remembered as:

"Control Spells Calm And Time To Treat"

and are listed in Box 13.1.

> **Box 13.1.** Incident officer priorities
>
> **C**ommand
> **S**afety
> **C**ommunications
> **A**ssessment
> **T**riage
> **T**reatment
> **T**ransport

Ambulance Incident Officer

The officer in charge of the ambulance resources at the scene is the Ambulance Incident Officer (AIO), who is not involved directly with patient care. The AIO is identified by a green and white chequered tabard, clearly labelled "AMBULANCE INCIDENT OFFICER." The AIO can move anywhere about the scene, but will usually stay close to the incident control vehicles and other incident officers at Silver command. The following are the AIO's duties:

- To liaise with the Medical Incident Officer, Police Incident Officer and Fire Incident Officer
- To delegate key tasks to other ambulance officers
- To ensure that there are adequate communications for all Health Service personnel
- To carry out an assessment of the scene
- To determine from where the Mobile Medical Teams are drawn
- To determine which hospitals will receive the casualties, in liaison with the Medical Incident Officer
- To establish primary triage
- To oversee ambulance treatment
- To organise the most suitable form of transport
- To confirm access and egress routes with the Police
- To determine the need for support from voluntary aid agencies and neighbouring Ambulance Services
- To arrange for replenishment of equipment
- To liaise with the Police regarding media briefings.

Understandably, there is considerable overlap between the duties of the Ambulance Incident Officer and those of the Medical Incident Officer. It is important from the outset that these two individuals function as a team. If they stay together efforts will not be duplicated, orders will not be contradictory, troublesome radio communications will be kept to a minimum, and difficult decisions will be shared.

Medical Incident Officer

The doctor in charge of the medical resources at the scene is the Medical Incident Officer (MIO) who is not involved with patient care. If this occurred it would compromise the MIO's ability to continue to control the overall scene. The MIO is identified by a green and white chequered tabard clearly labelled "MEDICAL INCIDENT OFFICER." This tabard will be available from the ambulance Emergency Control Vehicle. The MIO can move about the scene, but to be most effective he must work in close proximity to the Ambulance Incident Officer and other incident officers at Silver command. The following are the MIO's duties:

- To liaise with the Ambulance Incident Officer, Police Incident Officer, and Fire Incident Officer
- To delegate key tasks to other medical and nursing personnel
- To establish and maintain communications with senior personnel in receiving hospitals
- To carry out a medical assessment of the scene
- To establish specialist medical equipment needs and liaise with the Ambulance Service to obtain them
- To determine the need for medical and nursing personnel at the scene
- To determine which hospitals will receive casualties in liaison with the Ambulance Incident Officer

- To establish secondary triage
- To oversee treatment
- To liaise with the Police regarding media briefings.

The MIO's main task is to take control of the medical resources at the scene. All doctors and nurses arriving on scene must be tasked by the MIO, and on completion of specific tasks should report to the MIO for redeployment. A failure to enforce this will encourage Ambulance, Police, and Fire personnel to direct the doctors and nurses where they perceive the need: this will rapidly result in a loss of medical control and an inefficient service.

Although the MIO is responsible for the safety of medical personnel, the Ambulance Safety Officer has a specific role to identify hazards. To control medical resources effectively the MIO must establish communications with the Ambulance Emergency Control Vehicle and all the emergency service Incident Officers. This means physically finding the individual Incident Officers and speaking to them on arrival (they will usually be in the vicinity of the incident control vehicles). Poor liaison is common. The MIO must also make sure that medical and nursing personnel know and use the correct routes of communication.

An initial assessment of the scene, ideally made with the AIO, will help to determine the nature of the incident and the resources that are needed. The MIO is responsible for ensuring that triage is performed rapidly, accurately, and repeatedly, and will make sure that the best possible treatment is given to all casualties.

> **The Medical Incident Officer must *never* become involved with treating individual casualties**

The background of the individual performing the task of the Medical Incident Officer is less important than the fact that he has been adequately trained. It has been argued that the place for a single handed emergency medicine consultant is at the hospital, and that the job of Medical Incident Officer would be more appropriately done by a general practitioner, or another hospital doctor who is unlikely to be required in the immediate treatment phase. A general practitioner member of a local immediate care scheme is perhaps the most logical choice when available; these doctors are trained and equipped for pre-hospital work. The choice of MIO should therefore be from the following:

- Immediate care doctor, with additional major incident management training
- Senior accident and emergency medicine doctor, with additional pre-hospital and major incident management training, ideally not coming from the main receiving hospital
- Non-essential senior medical or surgical doctor with additional pre-hospital and major incident management training.

Nursing Incident Officer

When two or more medical teams containing nurses are present at the scene a Nursing Incident Officer (NIO) can be appointed. The NIO is identified by a green and white chequered tabard clearly labelled "NURSING INCIDENT OFFICER." This nurse is then responsible for determining the skill mix of the nurses present and assigning them to suitable treatment areas. It should be borne in mind that the nurses may have a diversity of backgrounds (including accident and emergency; surgery; intensive care; general ward work; and community), a range of experience (staff nurse, senior staff nurse, sister), and a difference in qualification (enrolled nurse, registered general nurse, or diploma).

The NIO must liaise closely with the MIO and AIO and should *not* be a member of any Mobile Medical Team. The NIO is not involved directly with patient care. To be most effective in this role the NIO should have received specialist training and be drawn from a bank of nurses known to have completed such training. Familiarity with working outside the hospital can be gained from experience in a "hospital flying squad" and will give this nurse the confidence and assertiveness needed in dealing with other members of the emergency services.

The NIO can be responsible for the allocation of controlled analgesic drugs to staff, keeping a signed record of the number of ampoules issued to each individual.

The NIO must be alert to individual fatigue among nursing staff and should brief the MIO of the continuing requirement for nurses at the scene.

AMBULANCE AND MEDICAL SERVICES' SITE PLAN

To understand how the Health Services work at the site, it is essential first to know the way in which the site is set out, and second to know the command structure that is necessary to oversee this. These two aspects of command and control are dealt with below.

Key locations

Figure 13.1 is a schematic representation of the key locations which are established by the Health Services during the onsite response.

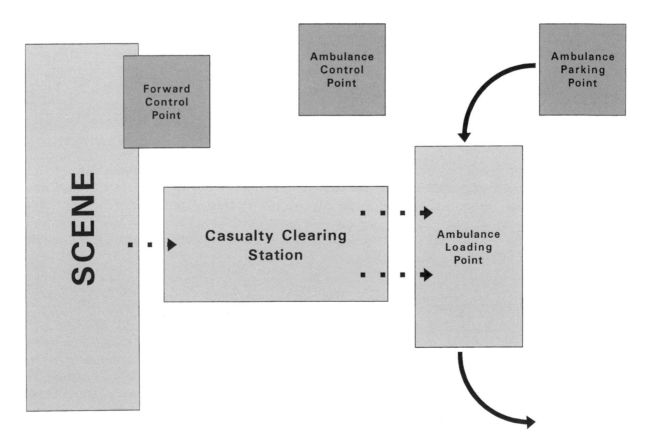

Figure 13.1. A schematic representation of the layout of the Health Services at a major incident

Each incident is different and the exact location of each area, and its relationship with other areas, will vary. It may even be necessary to leave some areas out altogether or to duplicate others; for example, if access to particular parts of the scene is difficult then two Casualty Clearing Stations might be set up with their associated Ambulance Loading Points.

Ambulance Control Point
This is usually in a mobile control vehicle and *should* be identified with a steady green light.

> **The Ambulance Control Point location is indicated by a steady green light**

It provides a focus for the deployment and control of Health Service resources, and may also provide an onsite communications facility.

> **All Health Service resources attending an incident must report to the Ambulance Control Point**

The control vehicle is usually parked close to the Police and Fire Command vehicles, to help scene coordination, but spaced 15 m apart to avoid radio interference.

Forward Control Point
This area is close to or within the immediate Bronze (operational) area of the incident, and is selected such that the Forward Incident Officers can direct operations using mobile communications. There may be a need to have more than one Forward Control Point to direct different sectors of a large scene.

Ambulance Parking Point
This is essentially a holding area where ambulances are kept until they are called forward to the Ambulance Loading Point. Ideally access, both from the arrival route and from the scene, should be good. In prolonged incidents this area becomes a focus for staff briefing, resupply, and refreshment.

Casualty Clearing Station
This area is set up by the Ambulance and Medical Incident Officers and serves as a focus for the triage sorting and treatment of casualties. The only absolute requirement is that this area should be safe. Access (both from the scene and to evacuation routes), shelter, light, and size also need to be considered. The Ambulance Loading Point (see below) is adjacent.

> **The Casualty Clearing Station is set up by the Ambulance and Medical Incident Officers after factors such as safety, access, shelter, and size have been considered**

When the Casualty Clearing Station is set up outside, areas for casualties of different priorities should be clearly marked. This may be done with different colour (red/yellow/ green) groundsheets, or separate inflatable tents. When tents are used they should not be crammed with stretcher patients—this simply takes the patient from one entrapment situation (the incident) into another (the tent). Close packing of stretchers allows little access to stretcher patients to treat them, or a flow of casualties through the area. Figure 13.2 is a representation of one layout of a Casualty Clearing Station which allows vertical and horizontal flow of casualties while awaiting evacuation: this "ideal" layout should serve as a framework for thought.

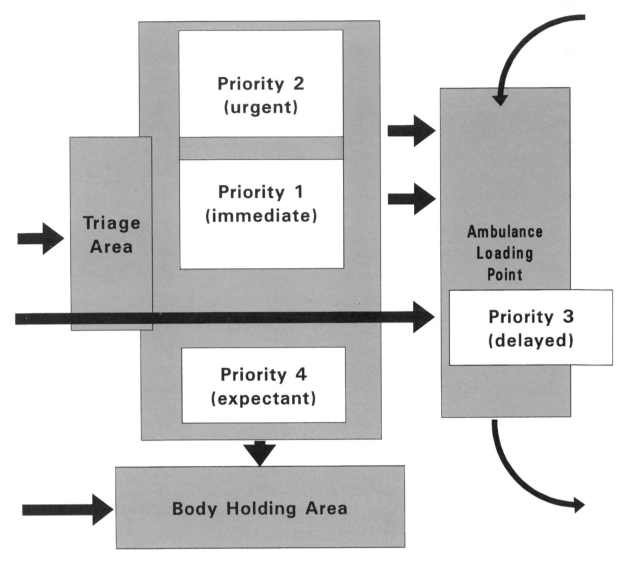

Figure 13.2. Schematic representation of a Casualty Clearing Station

Casualties can be moved inside the treatment areas, depending upon whether they improve or deteriorate. A similar movement should be possible within the evacuation area. This system will be able to allow for those whose priority changes during treatment or while waiting evacuation (see Chapter 18).

Ambulance Loading Point
This is the area where ambulances collect casualties from the Casualty Clearing Station for transportation to hospital.

Control of key areas

One of the most important steps in converting the chaos of a major incident into organised treatment is to establish control of the flow of patients. Equipment must be available to demarcate key areas and to signpost them. Plastic tape (green check to distinguish it from the blue and red tapes used by the Police and Fire Services respectively) can be used to control entry and exit points, and a large supply should be available. Collapsible signposts should be available to label the key areas. Some ambulance services have rapidly erectable tents which can provide a sheltered area for holding and treating casualties before transport.

AMBULANCE SERVICE COMMAND AND KEY ROLES

To facilitate the command and control of a major incident the Ambulance Service have adopted a standard structured "key role" approach. A number of specific roles have been identified, and these are filled by the initial crews arriving on the scene. Subsequently, the roles are handed on to more senior ambulance officers as they arrive.

This approach is flexible enough to allow most situations to be dealt with. Furthermore, the use of key roles rather than the specific appointment of officers to jobs avoids the problems that arise when particular officers are unavailable or cannot reach the scene.

Box 13.2. Ambulance Service key roles

First crew on scene
Ambulance Incident Officer
Forward Ambulance Incident Officer
Communications Officer—on site
Casualty Clearing Station Officer
Ambulance Loading Officer
Ambulance Safety Officer
Ambulance Parking Officer
Primary Triage Officer
Secondary Triage Officer

The key roles are listed in Box 13.2 and the command structure is shown in Figure 13.3.

First crew on scene

The first ambulance crew on the scene of a major incident will usually consist of a paramedic and a technician. Once it becomes apparent that a major incident has occurred the paramedic must assume the role of Ambulance Incident Officer until relieved by a more senior paramedic or ambulance officer. The first task is a scene assessment which should include the exact location, the type of incident, the hazards, and the numbers of casualties (including the presence of trapped patients). This information will allow early decisions about initial deployment of ambulances, equipment, and other resources (such as medical teams) to be made. It is absolutely vital that this crew does not get involved in patient management. This was discussed in more detail in Chapter 5.

Ambulance Safety Officer

This officer is responsible to the AIO for the health and safety of all Health Service personnel on site. He will report to the AIO. His duties are the following:

- To check that all Health Service personnel are wearing suitable protective clothing
- To monitor for fatigue or stress in staff and to advise on the need to evacuate staff

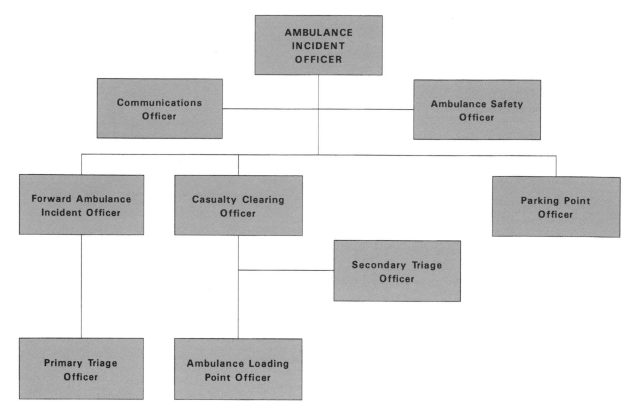

Figure 13.3. The Ambulance Service command and control structure

- To identify hazards and ensure that protective measures are taken
- To liaise with the other emergency services on safety matters and procedures
- To seek advice regarding the correct treatment procedures in cases of contamination of patients, staff, vehicles, or equipment.

Personnel who are not equipped with the correct protective clothing should be refused admission to the site

Communications Officer—on site

This officer provides and coordinates all onsite communications to ambulance officers and medical staff, and communications between the other emergency services. He works from the Ambulance Control Point (in the Emergency Control Vehicle). His duties are the following:

- To provide a link between the site and Central Ambulance Control
- To provide a link between the site Ambulance Emergency Control Vehicle and other emergency service incident control vehicles
- To provide a link between the site and the receiving hospitals
- To control the movement of ambulance vehicles on site
- To determine the most suitable communication mode for a particular message, including radio (VHF and UHF), telephone land lines, cellular telephone, and facsimile
- To record all the transmissions from the medical personnel at the site.

Forward Ambulance Incident Officer

This officer is responsible to the AIO for the management of ambulance resources. He works from the Forward Ambulance Control Point and is the eyes and ears of the AIO in the Bronze (operational) area of the incident. The following are his duties:

- To direct resources to deal with triage and removal of patients to the Casualty Clearing Station
- To determine the location of the Ambulance Parking Area and Loading Point.

Casualty Clearing Station Officer

In liaison with the Ambulance Incident Officer (and MIO if present) this officer will site the Casualty Clearing Station (CCS). When siting the CCS the following factors should be considered:

- The CCS should be a safe distance from all hazards
- Access to the CCS should not require long or difficult transport of patients from the incident site
- Natural shelter or buildings should be used when suitable
- There must be easy access for vehicles to load patients.

The first priority when setting up a CCS is to provide a treatment facility. This means picking a piece of ground and opening the treatment boxes or rucksacks. The establishment of this facility should not be delayed while waiting for tents to be put up.

The Casualty Clearing Station Officer will also do the following:

- Initiate and monitor the triage of casualties brought to the CCS
- Maintain records of patient movements
- In liaison with the doctor appointed in charge of the CCS, brief and monitor medical staff working in the CCS
- Ensure that there is adequate equipment within the CCS
- Liaise with the Ambulance Loading Officer for transportation needs and priorities of evacuation
- Keep the Ambulance Incident Officer updated of casualty numbers, severity, and movements.

Ambulance Loading Officer

This officer will work at the Ambulance Loading Point. His duties are the following:

- To liaise with the Police to ensure a suitable circuit of access and egress for ambulances (Figure 13.4)
- To ensure that casualties are transported in priority order
- To link with the Ambulance Parking Officer to ensure a steady flow of vehicles to the CCS
- To decide in consultation with the AIO and MIO the most appropriate form of transport (including commandeered public transport, fixed wing aircraft, helicopter, boat)
- To arrange the collection of all ambulance and medical equipment at the close of the incident and ensure that it is returned to its owner.

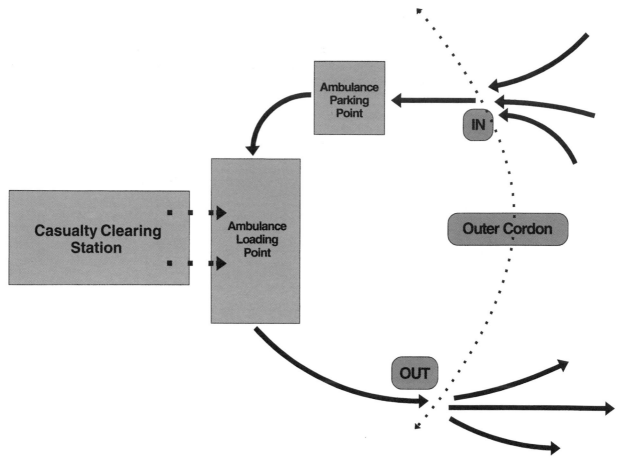

Figure 13.4. Ambulance vehicle circuit

Ambulance Parking Officer

This officer will work from the Ambulance Parking Point. The following are his duties:

- To ensure the best use of vehicular resources
- To maintain a log of staff and their vehicles attending the site
- To include in this log the qualifications of attending ambulance staff
- In conjunction with the AIO and FAIO, to send the appropriate ambulance personnel to the desired location
- To consider using ambulance care assistants for driving duties, thus releasing all qualified ambulance staff for patient treatment (in some circumstances traffic police officers may be used as ambulance drivers for the same reason).

Primary Triage Officer(s)

These officers supervise the triage of casualties at the point of first patient contact. They should carry out triage as discussed in Chapter 16, and label patients appropriately.

Equipment Officer

In addition to the above appointments it has usually been found necessary to appoint an Equipment Officer. This officer will oversee and distribute additional equipment brought to the scene. It is recommended that equipment is dispensed from one supply vehicle at a time, because the vehicle can then be taken away once it is depleted and can be completely replenished from a supply depot. A doctor or nurse may be appointed to assist at this supply dump when multiple Mobile Medical Teams attend and bring specialist equipment supplies with them.

MEDICAL COMMAND TASKS

The command tasks allocated to the medical services are shown in Figure 13.5. These can be seen to be complementary to those made by the Ambulance Service, and it is essential that medical service and Ambulance Service personnel liaise very closely during the response.

The particular tasks of the various appointees are shown below.

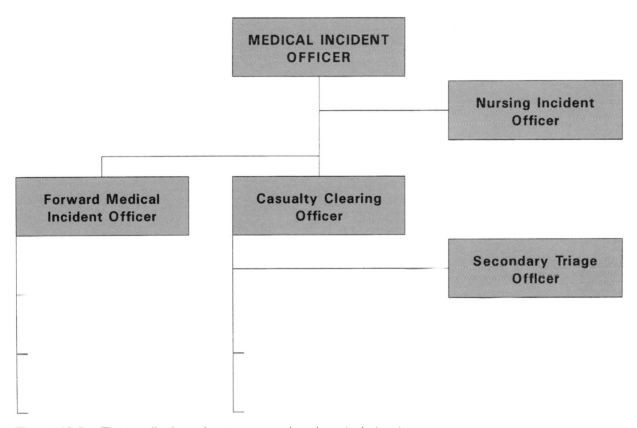

Figure 13.5. The medical services command and control structure

Forward Medical Incident Officer

This doctor is the eyes and ears of the MIO in the Bronze (operational) area. There should be no direct involvement with patient treatment.

The major task is supervision of the hospital teams and individual immediate care doctors arriving on the scene. Requests for a doctor or medical team to attend a casualty who is trapped must be directed from the attending paramedic through the FAIO to the FMIO and by no other route. It follows that the FMIO should work in close association with the FAIO.

Secondary Triage Officer

This doctor will be based in the CCS with the Casualty Clearing Station Officer. He should supervise the triage sort, and may be used to supervise some of the medical treatments in the CCS. Close liaison with the Ambulance Loading Officer is essential.

Team leaders

The team leader of each Mobile Medical Team or Mobile Surgical Team is directly responsible for the team's safety. This responsibility will have started in the hospital before leaving for the scene, and will end only after each team member has been debriefed both operationally and emotionally. Only the team leader should accept tasks, and team members should be given their tasks by their leader. The roles of the teams themselves are dealt with in more detail in Chapter 14.

Medical command and control at the scene can be complicated by the absence of a recognisable rank structure between hospital doctors and general practitioners who attend. The hierarchical hospital rank structure may well not be applicable to the scene, where training and ability are of paramount importance. This difficulty could be reduced if a system of pre-hospital training were adopted, and if the doctors working at the scene had helmet markings denoting their rank. Such a system is shown in Figure 13.6.

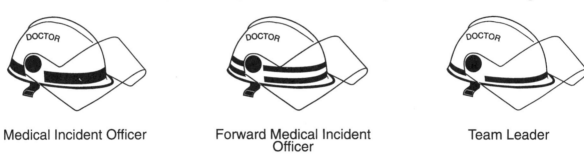

Medical Incident Officer   Forward Medical Incident Officer   Team Leader

Figure 13.6. Helmet markings for the medical services

Summary

- The Ambulance and Medical Incident Officers are in charge of the Health Services' response at the scene
- These two officers must liaise closely together
- The scene plan involves the setting up of two control points (one forward and one rear), a Casualty Clearing Station, and an Ambulance Loading Point
- To control and maintain the flow of ambulances for evacuation of casualties it is necessary to set up a circuit. An Ambulance Parking Point should be set up first
- The various areas set up by the Health Services are controlled by Ambulance, Medical, and Nursing Officers. Each officer must clearly understand his or her role if the plan is to work smoothly
- Ambulance personnel and medical teams will work within the various areas and will be under the command of the administrative officers in those areas

---

CHAPTER

14

Medical and nursing staff at the scene

After reading this chapter you should be able to answer the following questions:

- What medical and nursing staff will be at the scene?
- What teams could they belong to?
- What tasks could the various teams undertake?
- What are the priorities for these teams?

INTRODUCTION

The medical and nursing staff who attend a major incident form a small but highly skilled part of the Health Service response. It is essential that their skills are used effectively, and that they complement rather than challenge the role of ambulance technicians and paramedics.

Medical and nursing staff at the scene should complement rather than challenge the role of ambulance technicians and paramedics

As has been discussed earlier effective medical support requires good medical management, and to this end all medical and nursing staff must fit in to the Health Services' command and control structure discussed in Chapter 13. Teams must be properly equipped (both personally and medically), must be adequately experienced and skilled, and should be practised. If the teams fulfil these criteria, and are used correctly, the extra skills available will benefit the casualties immensely. If they are ill equipped, inexperienced, unskilled, or undisciplined then they become a liability not only to the casualties but also to the other rescuers.

MEDICAL AND NURSING STAFF AT THE SCENE

Medical and nursing staff will arrive at the scene either from the hospital or from the community. Those from the community may well be part of a local immediate care response system, whereas those from the hospital will usually have been mobilised from the receiving hospitals. Some health workers may become involved either because they are survivors of the incident, or because they were passing in the early stages. Whatever their origin, all staff need to be properly equipped and must report to the Ambulance Control Point for allocation of tasks by the MIO.

> **Health Service personnel who are inadequately equipped are unlikely to be allowed access to the site by the Ambulance Safety Officer**

Immediate care doctors

Most doctors who are part of an official immediate care response will arrive with both their personal and medical equipment. They are usually well trained and practised and have a high degree of local knowledge. They can therefore be allocated either command tasks or tasks concerned with patient assessment or care.

Hospital based teams

Teams that arrive from hospital have usually been summoned and transported by the Ambulance Service. Although all listed hospitals are required to provide a Mobile Medical Team (MMT), there is no official guidance regarding either the composition or equipment of the teams. The standard of preparation, equipment, and training is therefore variable.

Most hospitals will provide an MMT consisting of one or two doctors and the same number of nurses (Figure 14.1). It is not necessary for this team to have surgical expertise because the requirement for on scene surgery is small. Expertise in assessment and resuscitation is much more valuable, and in general this will mean that emergency department middle grade or senior doctors and nurses are involved.

Surgical input should be reserved for special cases, and should only be summoned at the request of the Medical Incident Officer. A Mobile Surgical Team (MST) consisting of one middle grade or senior surgeon, a similar grade of anaesthetist, and appropriate scrub and anaesthetic nurse support should be formed at a receiving hospital, and

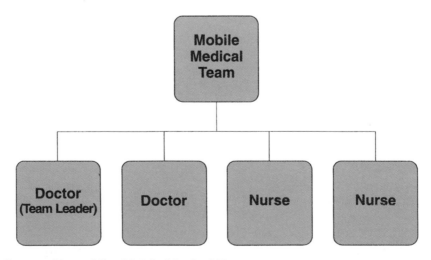

Figure 14.1. Composition of the Mobile Medical Team

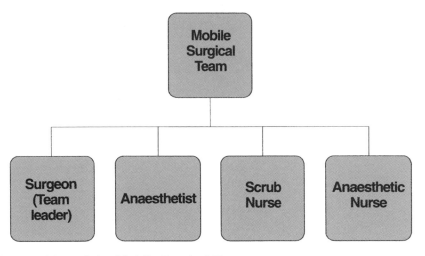

Figure 14.2. Composition of the Mobile Surgical Team

dispatched via ambulance to the scene (Figure 14.2). This team will work under the close supervision of an MMT.

Other health workers

Voluntary Aid Societies

Doctors and nurses who are members of the Voluntary Aid Societies may also be working at the scene. It is easy to let such staff function independently or within their own units, but close liaison with the unit commanders will ensure the most appropriate use of their skills.

Incidentally involved health workers

As mentioned above some doctors, nurses, and other health care staff may become involved at the scene by default. It is most unlikely that these staff will be equipped medically to provide anything more than basic first aid; furthermore their lack of proper personal protective equipment means that they are at considerable extra personal risk. The emergency service and medical staff who have been mobilised to the scene should therefore take over as soon as is possible. Health care staff who were involved in the incident should be treated as any other casualty, and those who have become involved incidentally should be given tasks away from the dangers of the scene itself.

> **Health workers who are not equipped for the scene can be deployed elsewhere**

Team tasks

Mobile Medical Team

The team may be broken up and allocated a number of command tasks, or may be kept together and allocated to an area. If they are allocated to the site of the incident they will be under the immediate control of the Forward Medical Incident Officer; if they are working in the Casualty Clearing Station they will be controlled by the Casualty Clearing Officer. As all incidents are different the exact nature of the team tasks and the priorities of these tasks will change. They are likely to include those shown in Box 14.1.

Box 14.1. Mobile Medical Team tasks

Triage at the site
Treatment of live casualties at the site
Triage in the Casualty Clearing Station
Treatment in the Casualty Clearing Station
Triage for transport
Treatment of casualties from other rescue services
Assistance to the Mobile Surgical Team if present
Assistance to the Ambulance Service in treatment of other minor injured people at the scene
Pronouncement and labelling of dead at the scene

Triage and treatment are dealt with in detail in Chapters 16 and 17 respectively.

Action cards can and should be used to specify who should be in the team, what immediate preparations are required, what equipment is needed (and where it can be found), how the team should move to the scene, and what their initial actions are on arrival. An example of the immediate actions specified on such a card is shown in Table 14.1.

Table 14.1. Immediate actions specified on a Mobile Medical Team action card

---

Immediate actions

1   On being nominated as a member of the Mobile Medical Team staff should proceed immediately to the accident and emergency department

2   Medical equipment and clothing should be collected from the major incident store. A nurse should obtain and sign for the major incident controlled drugs

3   Once an ambulance arrives to transport the team to the scene it should be loaded with all the major incident equipment except that for the Mobile Surgical Team

4   Having checked that no special orders for equipment have been asked for by the Medical Incident Officer, the Mobile Medical Team should proceed to the incident site in the ambulance

5   On arrival at the site all Mobile Medical Team personnel should report to the Medical Incident Officer at the Ambulance Control Point (usually indicated by a green steady light) for orders

6   Under the direction of the Medical Incident Officer undertake triage at the site using the following priorities:

    Priority 1—immediate
    Casualties requiring immediate life saving procedures

    Priority 2—urgent
    Casualties who will require surgery or other intervention within 6 hours

    Priority 3—delayed
    Less serious cases not requiring immediate treatment

    . . . and if it is considered necessary by the Medical Incident Officer:

    Priority 4—expectant
    Casualties whose injuries are so severe that they cannot survive in the circumstances

7   Under the direction of the Medical Incident Officer undertake treatment of casualties as necessary

---

Mobile Surgical Team

A Mobile Surgical Team should only be called to the scene of an incident by the Medical Incident Officer. This request should be task specific and will in general involve surgery for extrication. Very rarely other surgery that is life saving will be required.

The request for a Mobile Surgical Team should be task specific

It is essential that the Mobile Surgical Team is given the same standard of personal protective equipment as the MMT, and is instructed in its correct use. Once on scene the team should report to the Ambulance Control Point, and (because their pre-hospital training is likely to be minimal) must be accompanied and supervised throughout their stay. All or part of an MMT may be given this supervisory role, or ambulance staff may be allocated to oversee them.

As soon as the tasks that require surgical expertise are completed the team should be returned to the hospital that provided them, where their surgical skills can be used to the full.

Summary

- Medical and nursing staff at the scene of a major incident should be allowed to use their special skills to the full
- To achieve this, immediate care doctors and hospital based teams must be properly equipped, trained, and disciplined
- The exact nature and priority of tasks will vary with the incident. In general they will involve triage, treatment, and preparation for transport
- Surgical input at the scene should be limited, and should be task specific

CHAPTER

15

The hospital response

After reading this chapter you should be able to answer the following questions:

- Who is in charge of the Health Service response at the hospital?
- How is the hospital response organised?
- What are the roles of the accident and emergency staff?
- What are the roles of other hospital staff?

COMMAND AND CONTROL

The Health Service response at the hospital is controlled by the *Hospital Coordination Team* (as shown in Figure 15.1). The leader of this team is the *Medical Coordinator*, who

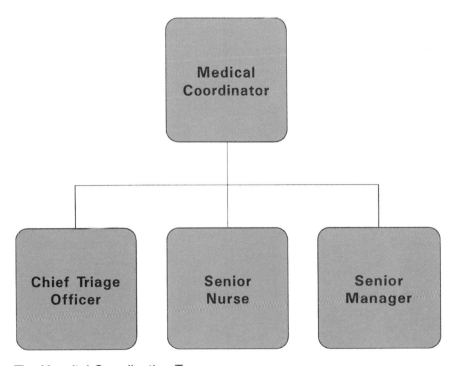

Figure 15.1. The Hospital Coordination Team

will usually be the medical director or his deputy. Also in this team are the *Chief Triage Officer*, a Senior Hospital Manager, and a Senior Nurse Manager.

> **The Health Service response at the hospital is controlled by the Hospital Coordination Team, which is led by the Medical Coordinator**

The Chief Triage Officer will be a Senior Emergency Physician, and is responsible for ensuring that the casualty reception area is prepared. This officer will perform the initial retriage of casualties on their arrival at the hospital, to determine which clinical area each patient is sent to.

KEY AREAS

The Senior Nurse Manager will ensure that the clinical areas are prepared to receive casualties, and will delegate the running of each area to a senior nurse. The key clinical areas are listed in Box 15.1.

> **Box 15.1.** Key clinical areas
>
> Triage
> Priority 1 (immediate) and 2 (urgent)
> Priority 3 (delayed)
> Preoperative and postoperative ward
> Admissions ward
> Operating rooms (theatres)
> Intensive care

The Senior Hospital Manager is responsible for coordinating the non-clinical areas and requirements. The key administrative areas and their use are listed in Box 15.2.

> **Box 15.2.** Key administrative areas
>
> | Key area | Use |
> |---|---|
> | Medical staff reporting | All doctors report here |
> | Nursing staff reporting | All nurses report here |
> | Volunteer reporting | Medical students + volunteers report here |
> | Hospital Information Centre | Information on all casualties, admitted or discharged, collated here |
> | Discharge and reunion area | Relatives/friends of those with minor injuries to wait here |
> | Bereaved relatives' area | Breaking of bad news and counselling |
> | Hospital enquiry point | Directed enquiries about patients to be made here |
> | Press room | Media briefed here |
> | Blood donation | If required |

CALL IN

Staff are called in using a cascade system; those key staff called first will then arrange for others from their department to be called. The switchboard will usually have the responsibility to alert the key staff, but this will be done by *appointment* rather than name—staff lists held for this reason must be kept up to date. Direct dial lines or public pay phones in each department should be used for the staff call in, thus avoiding the busy hospital switchboard. In some departments the cascade system is done by staff telephoning each other from home.

PREPARATION

Areas identified for immediate reception of casualties should be cleared as far as is practicable. Patients waiting for minor treatment in the emergency department should be advised to attend their general practitioner, or to attend a hospital distant from the incident. Wards designated as preoperative reception and postoperative recovery should be cleared. Inpatients in the designated wards should be discharged where appropriate, or moved to low dependency areas.

ACTION CARDS

On arriving at the hospital staff should attend the medical and nursing staff reporting points for task allocation. Those in key positions should be familiar with the hospital's Major Incident Plan and therefore aware of their initial responsibilities. Should this not be the case, and for the benefit of junior staff, *action cards* are distributed which briefly describe the duties of the individual. An example is given in Box 15.3. The action cards for key personnel will be part of the main hospital plan; those for junior members of staff may have to be prepared by individual departments.

TEAM ORGANISATION

The effective management of the hospital response is centred on the organisation of personnel into teams with specific tasks. These teams are the following:

- Casualty Treatment Teams
- Casualty Transfer Teams
- Operating Teams.

The Treatment and Transfer Teams are based in the initial treatment areas in and around the accident and emergency department. These teams are controlled by the *Team Coordinator*, who is a senior member of staff appointed by the Medical Coordinator. The Team Coordinator will be located in the reception area and will form medical and nursing staff into these teams as the staff become available.

TREATMENT

In a major incident there will be surgical and medical casualties. The proportions will depend upon the nature of the incident. A bomb, for example, will produce multiple surgical patients, whereas a crowd crush will produce multiple patients requiring cardiopulmonary resuscitation. Team composition will have to reflect this. The clinical activity in each area will be controlled by a triage officer who is responsible to the Chief Triage Officer. In the Priority 1 (immediate) area there will be a Surgical Triage Officer (usually the duty consultant surgeon), and a Medical Triage Officer (either a consultant physician or intensive care specialist), who will direct the treatment and transfer teams; these officers will also supervise treatment within the Priority 2 (urgent) area. Triage

Box 15.3. Example of an action card

Chief Triage Officer

Responsibilities
1   Overall control of the reception areas
2   Staffing of key appointments in the reception areas
3   Control of initial reception and management
4   Initial triage of major incident casualties
5   Assistance to the Medical Coordinator after the reception phase has ended
6   Operational debriefing of accident and emergency (A&E) medical staff involved in the major incident response

Immediate action
1   Assume control of the reception areas
2   Ensure that the preparation of the reception areas is complete
3   Ensure that the following posts are filled:
    Surgical Triage Officer
    Medical Triage Officer
    Surgical Triage Registrar
    Medical Triage Registrar
    If not appoint suitably senior doctors until the key personnel arrive
4   Assess the number of Casualty Treatment Teams required immediately in the reception areas and inform the Medical Coordinator
5   Triage major incident casualties as follows:
    Priority 1 (immediate)
    Casualties requiring immediate life saving procedures
    Priority 2 (urgent)
    Casualties who will require surgery or other intervention within 6 hours
    Priority 3 (delayed)
    Less serious cases not requiring immediate treatment
6   Continue to assess the situation and if necessary establish a further priority as follows:
    Priority 4 (expectant)
    Casualties whose injuries are so severe that they cannot survive in the circumstances
7   As further Casualty Treatment Teams are required inform the Medical Coordinator
8   As Casualty Transfer Teams are required inform the Medical Coordinator
9   Liaise with the Senior A&E Nurse regarding senior nurse staffing and supplies in the reception areas
10 Liaise with the Senior A&E Duty Clerk regarding documentation in the reception areas
11 Constantly monitor the triage, treatment, staffing, documentation, and supplies in the reception areas
12 Once the reception phase is over assist the Medical Coordinator to control the hospital response

Priorities during the incident
1   Overall control of the reception areas
2   Triage in the reception areas
3   Control of staffing in the reception areas
4   Control of treatment in the reception areas
5   Control of documentation in the reception areas
6   Control of supplies in the reception areas
7   Assisting the Medical Coordinator to control the hospital response

An effective hospital response is centred around forming personnel into treatment, transfer, and operating teams

responsibilities in the Priority 3 (delayed) area can be delegated to the surgical triage *registrar* and the medical triage *registrar.*

The Surgical Triage Officer will ensure that the highest priority surgical casualties are transferred directly to the operating rooms/theatres, but once the capacity of these is reached then further casualties will wait for surgery on the preoperative ward. The Surgical Triage Officer will also appoint a medical deputy to oversee activity in the operating theatres (*Senior Surgeon, Theatres*), and on the preoperative ward (*Senior Surgeon, Preop*). Specifically, the Senior Surgeon in Theatres will coordinate the Operating Teams and any specialist surgeons needed for particular procedures; the Senior Surgeon in Preop will coordinate the Treatment Teams on the preoperative ward. Both will keep the Surgical Triage Officer informed of surgical matters in their areas.

The Senior Nurse Manager will nominate a deputy (*Senior Nurse, Theatres*; *Senior Nurse, Preop*) who is responsible for ensuring that the preoperative and surgical areas are adequately prepared and staffed to receive casualties. Following surgery casualties will be transferred back to the preoperative/postoperative ward, but if this is full then a postoperative overflow ward will be established. In hospitals where the accident and emergency department has a "short stay" ward, then this ward is ideal to be designated as the preoperative/postoperative ward, because it can usually be cleared rapidly in the event of a major incident; the overflow ward would then be in the main hospital.

The Medical Triage Officer will direct the transfer of the most seriously ill patients to the intensive care unit. The duty intensive care consultant will assess the bed availability in his own and surrounding hospitals; when his own unit is full, he will discuss the transfer of patients to other hospitals' intensive care units with the Medical Coordinator. The Senior Nurse Manager will nominate a deputy (*Senior Nurse, Intensive Care*) who is responsible for preparing and staffing the intensive care unit.

Those casualties who do not require immediate surgery or intensive care facilities will be transferred to the admissions ward. This ward will be supervised by the Medical Triage Officer, and staffed by Treatment Teams that the Team Coordinator will nominate. The preparation of this ward will be delegated to a senior nurse (*Senior Nurse, Admissions*).

STAFF RESPONSIBILITIES

Accident and emergency

The procedures for declaring a major incident, and the immediate actions of the accident and emergency staff on receiving a major incident alert message, have been described earlier. It is worth restating that, if a major incident has not been recognised by the Ambulance Service and declared at the scene, or if casualties arrive by self evacuation at a nearby hospital very rapidly after the incident, then the accident and emergency department must declare a major incident. In some instances it may be necessary only to activate a limited response of additional accident and emergency (A&E) staff—this would be done by the duty A&E consultant.

Many medical and nursing staff who are assigned to work in the treatment and transfer teams, based in accident and emergency, will be unfamiliar with the detailed layout of the department, and particularly with where equipment can be found. For this reason it is important to identify regular A&E staff with a tabard.

Most A&E staff will form into treatment teams to work in the high dependency areas (immediate and urgent Priorities) within the department.

Other departments

Each department is responsible for maintaining an up to date list of its doctors and nurses who can be called in from home (if off duty) in the event of a major incident.

The junior medical staff resident within the hospital can by alerted by tannoy or pager and initially can institute the call in of their seniors who are *on duty* at home. A member of staff can then be nominated to call those who are off duty, using a cascade system.

When staff arrive at the hospital it is important that they do not simply go to their ward or department, but that they attend the medical or nursing staff reporting points. Here they will be logged and senior personnel can be allocated key administrative roles if these are unfilled. Tabards and action cards will be issued and staff directed to the Team Coordinator for allocation to a Treatment or Transfer Team, or to the Surgical Triage Officer for allocation to an Operating Team.

Transfer Teams are required to look after those patients moving from the high dependency areas (Priority 1 and Priority 2) to the operating rooms, preoperative ward, or intensive care unit. Additionally, teams may be necessary for the secondary transfer of patients, for example, to a neighbouring hospital's intensive care unit. In this case it will be important to have a doctor with anaesthetic experience and a nurse experienced in the use of a portable ventilator and anaesthetic/resuscitation drugs. Care must be taken to use skilled personnel appropriately for treatment or transfers, and identify those with extended training (Advanced Trauma Life Support, Advanced Cardiac Life Support, Advanced Paediatric Life Support) to work in the high dependency areas.

DOCUMENTATION

At the scene the casualties will have triage labels attached to them. If they are evacuated rapidly it is likely that very little, if any, information will be recorded. Those casualties who have been trapped at the scene or received treatment in the Casualty Clearing Station may, however, have important clinical details regarding injuries, treatment, and serial observations recorded on this label. It is therefore important that, if new documentation is instituted at the hospital, the pre-hospital data are not removed, but kept with the patient.

In the initial reception area each patient will be issued with a major incident casualty card and given a wrist band with the corresponding number, which must not be removed under any circumstances. The senior nurse in each of the treatment areas is responsible for completing a casualty statement form at regular intervals and returning this to the Hospital Information Centre: the admissions officer can then maintain an accurate casualty state board.

Summary
- The Health Service response at the hospital is controlled by the Hospital Coordination Team, led by the Medical Coordinator
- The effective management of the hospital response is dependent on the organisation of personnel into Treatment, Transfer, and Operating Teams
- A major incident can involve medical as well as surgical casualties. Within the treatment areas priorities are determined by the Surgical Triage Officer and the Medical Triage Officer

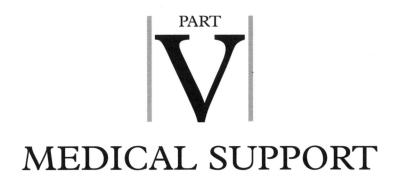

MEDICAL SUPPORT

CHAPTER

16

Triage

After reading this chapter you should be able to answer the following questions:

- What is triage?
- When is triage carried out?
- Where is triage carried out?
- What priorities should be used?
- How are priorities assigned?
- What casualty labels should be applied?

HISTORY

Triage, meaning to sieve or to sort, is the first step in the hierarchy of *medical support* at major incidents.

Box 16.1 The hierarchy of medical support

Triage
Treatment
Transport

Triage was first described by Surgeon Marshall Dominique Jean Larrey who was Napoleon's chief medical officer. He introduced a system of sorting the casualties who presented to the field dressing stations. His aims were military rather than medical—and highest priority was given to soldiers who had minor wounds and who could therefore be returned quickly to the line with minimum treatment. There is no English language record of the use of triage until the First World War. The official history of the United States Army in this conflict uses the word triage when describing the physical area where sorting was done, rather than a description of the sorting itself. Triage has continued since then to be the cornerstone of military medicine and has, in fairly recent times, been formally adopted in the management of most civilian emergency departments.

113

AIMS

The aims of triage, wherever it is done, are not only to deliver the right patient to the right place at the right time so that they receive the optimum treatment, but also to "do the most for the most," accepting that valuable medical resources should not be diverted to treating an irrecoverable condition. It can be deduced from this that triage principles should be applied whenever the number of casualties exceeds the skilled help immediately available.

> **Triage principles should be used whenever the number of casualties exceeds the number of skilled rescuers available**

Thus triage should take place during the management of emergencies ranging from road traffic accidents (where there might be four or five casualties and only one or two paramedics in attendance), to major incidents where, in spite of large numbers of medical, nursing, and paramedical staff, the number of casualties is so large that decisions about the order of their care needs to be taken.

TIMING

Triage is a dynamic rather than a static process. The state of the patient may change for the better or worse either because of a progression of the injuries, or as a result of interventions that are made.

> **Triage is a dynamic (continuous) process**

Triage must therefore be repeated many times during the care of a casualty. For example, a typical casualty might undergo triage: when he is first seen; before movement from the immediate scene debris; in the Casualty Clearing Station; before evacuation; on reception in hospital; during resuscitation and treatment; and before surgery. In addition to these occasions (which correspond to events external to the patient), a reassessment of priority will be necessary whenever the patient's condition is noted to have changed.

SITE

The first triage decision (the *triage sieve*) tends to be undertaken at the place where the casualty is found. Subsequent decisions at the scene (the *triage sort*) are taken at the Casualty Clearing Station (which is sited by agreement between the Ambulance and Medical Incident Officers as discussed in Chapter 13). Many Ambulance Services, and some known high risk areas such as airports, now have portable inflatable shelters

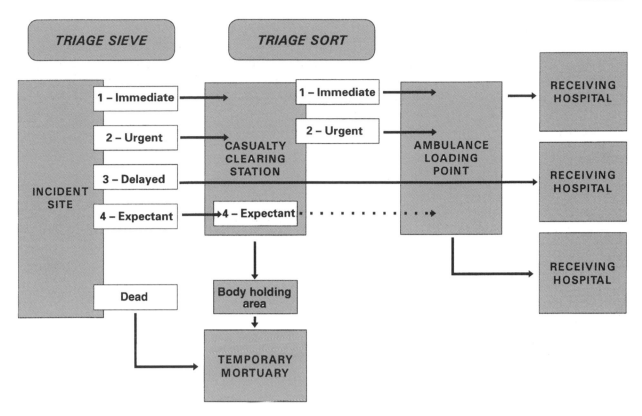

Figure 16.1. Triage and evacuation map

which can be used to form the Casualty Clearing Station. A schematic triage and evacuation map is shown in Figure 16.1.

In this scheme it is envisaged that triage on the scene will be carried out either by ambulance officers/paramedics or doctors, whereas that in the Casualty Clearing Station would be carried out by a doctor. Some patients such as the minor injured, may bypass the second triage stage and move directly via the evacuation area to a receiving hospital.

PRIORITIES

As mentioned above the aim of triage is to sort patients in such a way that it becomes possible to deliver the right patient to the right place at the right time. As a first step towards achieving this, patients are assigned to different priority groups.

Two systems of priorities are widely used in civilian practice. They are commonly referred to as the "P" (priority) system and the "T" (treatment) system and are illustrated in Table 16.1.

Table 16.1. Triage priorities

"P"	"T"	Description	Colour
1	1	Immediate	Red
2	2	Urgent	Yellow
3	3	Delayed	Green
	4	Expectant	Blue
Dead	Dead	Dead	White

The major difference between the two systems can be seen to be the inclusion of a fourth (expectant) category in the "T" system. For the purposes of this text the T system will be used. The four priority groups are defined as shown below.

Priority 1 (immediate)—Casualties who require immediate life saving procedures.

Priority 2 (urgent)—Casualties who require intervention within 4–6 hours.

Priority 3 (delayed)—Less serious cases who do not require treatment within the times given above.

Priority 4 (expectant)—Casualties whose injuries are so severe that they either cannot survive in the circumstances or would require so much input from the limited resources available that their treatment would seriously compromise the treatment of large numbers of other less seriously ill casualties.

Whether or not the last category has to be established is very much a decision for the Ambulance and Medical Incident Officers, and depends on resources available at the scene, the speed of evacuation, and the resources available in hospital. It may also be necessary to establish this category within a hospital if the resources available to treat the casualties are inadequate, and this again is a decision that should be made at the highest level.

> **Avoiding the use of the Priority 4 (expectant) category may cost lives**

The overvigorous avoidance of the use of this category is probably a mistake, because failure to use it correctly will in fact cost lives rather than save them.

It is essential that all the health care providers who attend a major incident use both the same priority groups and the same criteria for categorising patients into these groups. In the past different organisations have used different words to describe priorities, different colours to signify them, and widely differing triage criteria. This can lead to considerable confusion both at the scene and subsequently in receiving hospitals. It is recognised, however, that many triage labelling systems do not include an expectant label—in these circumstances use the Priority 3 (delayed) category, but separate them from the "walking wounded."

SORTING

Having decided what priorities to use to sort the patients the exact methods of sorting them must be established. For the first person on the scene this represents a considerable problem. There may be huge numbers of casualties and therefore a huge number of critical decisions that need to be made very quickly. "First look" triage (that carried out by the first rescuers on the scene as a quick assessment of the casualties) therefore needs to be rapid, simple, safe, and reproducible.

> **Initial triage decisions need to be made quickly, safely, and reproducibly**

Once this first look triage has been carried out, more time will be available for a more detailed assessment. These two stages of the triage process will be referred to as the "triage sieve" and the "triage sort" respectively.

Triage sieve

This stage of triage (first look) quickly sorts the casualties into priorities. As it is quick it is not perfect; however, any mistakes made at this stage can be corrected later on.

Mobility

Casualties who can still walk are the most easy to categorise. They are all assigned to Priority 3 (delayed) and can be shepherded from the site. This is referred to as the mobility sieve.

Walking patients are initially categorised as Priority 3 (delayed)

The astute may argue that it is possible to walk with a knife sticking our of your back or with 50% burns; eventually such patients will collapse and because triage is dynamic their priority will then change. Remember, the triage sieve is no more than a snapshot of the patient at an instant in time, not a predictor of what might develop later. That is why triage must be dynamic.

ABC

Those patients who are not walking will be initially categorised as either Priority 1 (immediate) or Priority 2 (urgent). They are sorted according to the airway, breathing, and circulatory (ABC) parameters described below.

Airway patency is assessed by performing a simple opening manoeuvre (chin lift and jaw thrust) if necessary, and assessing whether or not breathing occurs. Those patients who cannot breathe in spite of this manoeuvre are dead.

**Patients who cannot breathe in spite of simple airway
manoeuvres are dead**

Those who can breathe can proceed to the second assessment which is of respiratory rate. If the respiratory rate is unusually low (<10) or unusually high (>29) then the casualty is assigned to the Priority 1 (immediate).

If the rate is normal (between 10 and 29 breaths/min), then an assessment of circulation is carried out.

**Casualties with respiratory rates $\geqslant 30$ or $\leqslant 10$ breaths/min
are Priority 1 (immediate)**

The circulatory assessment is difficult even within hospital, and is even more so in the pre-hospital environment. Capillary refill time is assessed in the nail bed. If it is more than two seconds then the patient is assigned to Priority 1 (immediate). Obviously external exsanguinating haemorrhage should be stopped at this stage. If capillary refill is less than two seconds then the patient is assigned to the Priority 2 (urgent).

117

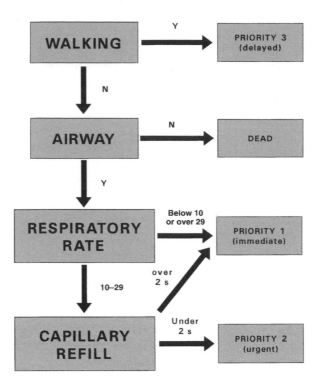

Figure 16.2. The triage sieve

**Casualties with a capillary refill time of more than two seconds
are Priority 1 (immediate)**

Capillary refill time is used for the circulatory assessment because it can be ascertained rapidly and reflects peripheral tissue perfusion. It is, however, affected by ambient temperature, and will be significantly reduced in normal subjects in cold conditions. It is reasonable to assume that the normal capillary refill time for a casualty is the same as that for a rescuer when in the same conditions. Thus in cold weather rescuers should be aware of their own capillary refill time and adjust the triage sieve accordingly. In extremely cold conditions the capillary refill time may become impossible to use and in such circumstances it is reasonable to use a pulse of 120 beats/min as the circulatory sieve, but this will take longer to assess (a capillary refill takes seven seconds—five seconds to press and two seconds to read; a pulse takes about 15 seconds to take).

The airway, breathing, and circulatory aspect of the triage sieve is illustrated in Figure 16.2.

**In cold conditions the circulatory assessment will need to be adjusted,
and in extreme conditions it may be replaced
by an assessment of the pulse rate**

Once the triage sieve has been carried out each of the patients will have been allocated to a triage category. This will allow rescuers who arrive later to go straight to the "immediate" priority patients, and treat and transport them first. It is probable that the triage will be carried out at the site of the incident; the categories assigned at that time will be used to move the patients from the site to the Casualty Clearing Station.

Triage sort

Once patients arrive in the Casualty Clearing Station they can be retriaged in a more leisurely manner. This process is termed the "triage sort."

In broad terms there are two approaches. The first is anatomical: when using this method all the injuries are identified and an overall picture of the urgency of the patient is gained. The patient is then placed into a triage category according to this assessment.

> **Anatomical methods of triage require a full secondary survey**

Although this is the gold standard against which all other methods of triage are measured it is in fact impractical in a pre-hospital setting. In particular it requires a full secondary survey which would necessitate the patient being fully undressed; it also requires a wide medical knowledge so that each of the injuries discovered can first be assigned an individual urgency, and then be grouped together to give an overall urgency for the patient. Finally it is extremely time consuming in the mass casualty situation.

An alternative method is the physiological approach. In this method the description is not of the injuries themselves but of their physiological consequence. Many scoring systems have been described, and the best known of these is probably the Trauma Score.

In the pre-hospital setting the Triage Revised Trauma Score (TRTS) has been advocated as the best system currently available. This is based on just three parameters as shown in Table 16.2.

Table 16.2. Triage Revised Trauma Score parameters

Parameter	Coded value
Respiratory rate	0–4
Systolic blood pressure	0–4
Glasgow coma scale	0–4

These parameters are coded as shown in Table 16.3, to give a score from 0 to 12.

The TRTS can thus be used to assign triage priorities as shown in Table 16.4.

If Priority 4 (expectant) is in use then a TRTS of 1–3 should be used to define it.

Work carried out for the US Navy has shown that non-expert staff can provide reliable trauma scores for casualties after a very short period of training. The use of such a scoring system is therefore feasible. Furthermore, many modern casualty labels (see below) incorporate trauma scoring as part of the patient report.

The advantages of the physiological methods are that they are quick, reproducible, and essentially merely an extension of the triage sieve. They do not, however, take into account the nature of the injury at all, and therefore cannot be used to decide whether a patient should be dispatched to a specialist or a general facility.

By mixing together the best parts of the anatomical and physiological methods discussed above, something close to the ideal can be achieved. The rapidity and simplicity of a physiological method such as the TRTS are used to define the initial priority. This is supplemented by as much relevant anatomical information as can be obtained in the time and conditions. Thus patients with head injury can be selected for neurosurgical centres, and patients with burn injury can be sent to regional burns centres. If evacuation is delayed, the anatomical information can be expanded up to the level of a full secondary survey as time allows.

The recommended method of assigning priorities is as follows:

Table 16.3. Triage Revised Trauma scoring system

Physiological variable	Measured value	Score
Respiratory rate	10–29	4
	>29	3
	6–9	2
	1–5	1
	0	0
Systolic blood pressure	$\geqslant$90	4
	76–89	3
	50–75	2
	1–49	1
	0	0
Glasgow coma scale	13–15	4
	9–12	3
	6–8	2
	4–5	1
	3	0

Table 16.4. Triage Revised Trauma Score and priority

Priority	TRTS
T1	1–10
T2	11
T3	12
Dead	0

The first look triage assessment is carried out at the site of injury by using the triage sieve; this is followed (usually in the Casualty Clearing Station) by a mixed approach to triage sorting—consisting of a physiological score (such as the TRTS) supplemented by relevant anatomical information.

Physiological methods of triage should be used first. These can be supplemented by as much anatomical information as time and conditions allow

TRIAGE LABELLING

There is little point in triaging casualties into priorities if other rescuers are not made aware of the results of the assessment. Some form of labelling is necessary. To be maximally effective a triage label should be highly visible, should use the standard categories (numbers, words, and colours) discussed above, and should be easily and firmly secured to the patient. It must also allow the patient's priority to be altered as the condition changes.

120

Triage labels must be highly visible, easily and securely attached,
and allow for priorities to be changed

It is helpful if the triage labels themselves can be used for making other clinical notes in the field. In general the primary colours are preferred because these show up better under difficult ambient lighting conditions. The labelling of the dead is important; the dead label can either be part of the standard triage label or may be a special card designed for this purpose. This is discussed further in Chapter 19.

Types

In broad terms two types of triage label exist—single and cruciform.

Single

When using the single triage label, a label marked with the appropriate priority is attached to the patient; these labels generally consist of a piece of coloured card with printed headings and space for patient information. The single label system is illustrated in Figure 16.3. As a single coloured card is attached to the patient, changing between categories is relatively difficult because the first card must be removed before the new card is attached. This is doubly disadvantageous if notes about the patient have been made on the first card because either this card must be left in place, or the notes that have been made on it must be transferred to the new card. If the first card is left then confusion can arise about the current category of the patient.

Single card triage labelling systems are not ideal for dynamic triage

In general, single label cards are poor if dynamic triage is to be carried out. A variation on the single label card is the *Mettag* label. This consists of a single label which has a number of colour coded perforated strips on its bottom edge; each strip accords to a

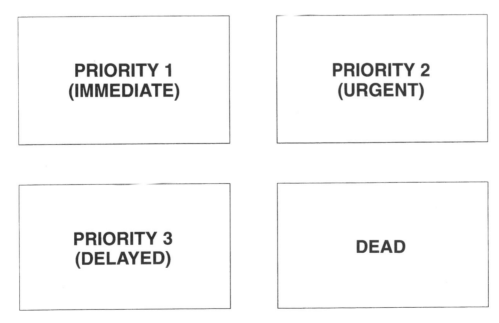

**PRIORITY 1
(IMMEDIATE)**

**PRIORITY 2
(URGENT)**

**PRIORITY 3
(DELAYED)**

DEAD

Figure 16.3. Single label system

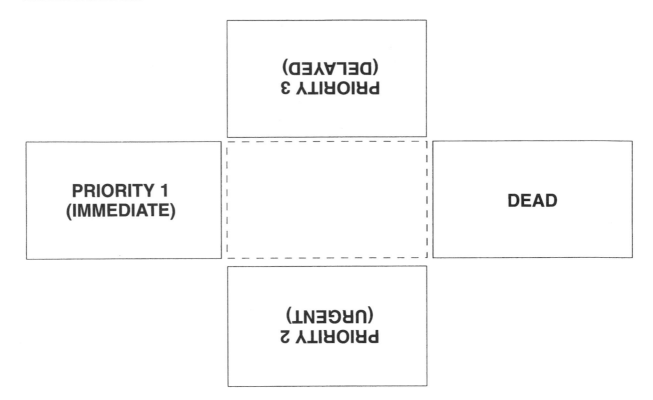

Figure 16.4. Cruciform label system

different triage category. The strips that do not apply to the patient are removed by the rescuer performing triage—and the lowest strip remaining therefore corresponds to the patient's priority. This card has two disadvantages: first, if the patient gets better then it is necessary either to replace the card or to stick the strips that have been torn off back on (that is, the patient can only deteriorate dynamically); second, the strip on the card designating the priority is not large, and is therefore not visible from a distance. This makes it difficult for a triage officer, or another rescuer, to look around and assess the number of patients in a particular category in a particular area.

Cruciform

The second general approach is the use of a cruciform card. These cards, as their name suggests, are shaped like a cross. When all the corners of the cross are folded into the middle they become rectangular. This is illustrated in Figure 16.4.

> **Cruciform triage labels can be used from the time of first triage on the scene to final triage in the receiving hospital**

The cards are folded in such a way that only the desired one of the four priorities is left on the outside; if the priority is changed then it is a simple matter to refold the card and show the new priority on the outside. This system overcomes the problem of additional data because the same card can be used however many times the priority is changed.

These cards are extremely useful for dynamic triage, but of course can be abused by the casualties themselves who may refold them to give themselves a higher priority.

Although triage labelling is essential, it is not always necessary to use the complex triage cards discussed above. Coloured pegs, corresponding to the triage category, are quite adequate during the first look triage (triage sieve), and are easily carried on the belt of a rescuer's clothing.

**Simple alternatives such as the use of coloured pegs
are acceptable during the triage sieve**

PERSONNEL

Triage is an essential but difficult task. It should always be carried out by the most senior and experienced person present, and thus over the course of an incident the person doing the triage may change from an ambulance paramedic to a senior clinician. Whoever does it, the principles are the same.

Summary
- Triage is the first step in the hierarchy of medical support at a major incident
- It is a dynamic process, starting with a triage sieve at the site where the casualties are found, moving via a physiological and anatomical triage sorting process in the Casualty Clearing Station, and continuing in the receiving hospitals to the point of definitive care
- Cruciform labels are the best available for dynamic triage

CHAPTER
17
Treatment

After reading this chapter you should be able to answer the following questions:

- Where is treatment carried out on the scene?
- How much treatment is carried out?
- What treatments are carried out?
- Who carries out the treatment?

INTRODUCTION

During a major incident a great many people will become involved in giving treatment to the injured and ill. These people will range in experience from the concerned bystander to the advanced life support provider.

Initial treatment (that given in the first few minutes after an incident) is usually delivered by other survivors (who may themselves be injured) and bystanders who were close to the incident when it occurred. Some of those providing this immediate treatment may be trained in basic first aid, and will therefore be able to provide a slightly more structured form of care. This first aid may be life saving.

Initial first aid will be provided by other survivors and bystanders

---

It is only when the emergency services begin to arrive that large numbers of people trained in first aid are likely to be found on the scene. All Police and Fire Service personnel receive instruction in life saving first aid; furthermore, the Fire Service carry some advanced life support equipment (a variable amount) and have firefighters trained to use it. Once their initial responsibilities have been discharged both these services will become involved in early treatment.

Once their initial tasks have been accomplished both the Police and Fire Services can assist in basic treatment

---

The Ambulance Service have overall responsibility for providing treatment at all incidents outside hospital. The skills of individuals within this service range from life saving first aid by ambulance auxiliaries to advanced life support by paramedics. The ambulance service input will be supplemented by the doctors and nurses sent to the scene either from immediate care schemes or as Mobile Medical Teams.

Box 17.1. The hierarchy of medical support

Triage
Treatment
Transport

It is absolutely essential that those managing the Health Service response remember the hierarchy of medical support as shown in Box 17.1. To achieve the best overall outcome for the casualties, triage must precede both treatment and transport. Once triage has been carried out the limited advanced treatment capability can be directed to those casualties who have the greatest need. Rescuers with a lower skill level can be used to look after casualties with less demanding problems.

WHERE IS TREATMENT CARRIED OUT?

The vast majority of first aid measures by bystanders will occur at the site of an incident. These procedures (which are unlikely to involve airway and breathing manoeuvres) will be carried out within the first few minutes after an incident has occurred. Once the emergency services arrive and the Health Services' command and control structure is in place, the focus of advanced activity is likely to move to the Casualty Clearing Station. Figure 17.1 summarises this.

Casualties who are entrapped may clearly need advanced life support procedures and these will have to be delivered at the site. Similarly, casualties who arrive at the Casualty Clearing Station requiring only first aid will not be returned to the scene but will be treated there.

Packaging for transfer is carried out in the Casualty Clearing Station, usually in an area adjacent to the Ambulance Loading Point.

HOW MUCH TREATMENT?

The aim of treatment at the scene of an incident is not to return the casualties to health, but to ensure that they are well enough to endure the journey to a facility where they can be fully assessed and treated.

Triage and treatment are heavily intertwined. The priority that patients are given will be reflected to a large degree by how much treatment they receive at the scene. Thus a walking patient who has been categorised Priority 3 (delayed) will most probably be moved to a hospital without receiving any treatment at all. On the other hand, a casualty with a compromised airway who has been categorised Priority 1 (immediate) may well require considerable input at the scene, so as to make transportation safe.

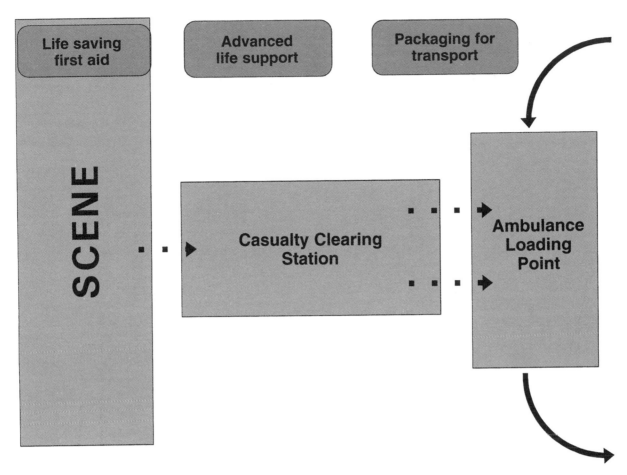

Figure 17.1. Treatment at the scene

> The aim of treatment at the scene is to allow the casualty to reach hospital safely

> The amount of treatment delivered at the scene corresponds to the triage priority

WHAT TREATMENT?

Virtually any treatment *can* be carried out in the pre-hospital setting. This fact alone does not mean that all treatments *should* be provided at the scene of a major incident. The aim of treatment remains the safe transportation of the casualty to hospital; thus the amount of treatment carried out should be limited to that which ensures that this is possible.

Overall medical management will be optimal if treatment is kept at this level. If too little is done patients will die unnecessarily on the way to hospital. If too much is done then time that could have been spent with other patients will have been wasted.

Treatments at the scene are therefore likely to be confined to those concerned with problems of the airway, breathing, and circulation. In addition, advanced life support measures to prevent exacerbation of spinal injuries will form an integral part of packaging

127

for transfer. Although other treatments (up to and including amputation for extrication) may be required on occasion, these will be rare.

Most treatment at a major incident will be directed towards the airway, breathing, and circulation

---

The range of clinical skills that may be needed at the major incident scene are shown in Table 17.1.

Table 17.1. Basic and advanced treatments

	Basic	Advanced
Airway	Airway opening ● Chin lift ● Jaw thrust	Oropharyngeal airway Nasopharyngeal airway Oral tracheal intubation Surgical airway ● Needle cricothyroidotomy ● Surgical cricothyroidotomy
Spinal control	Manual cervical stabilisation	Logrolling Cervical collar application Spinal board application Rapid extrication
Breathing	Mouth to mouth ventilation Mouth to nose ventilation	Mouth to mask ventilation Bag–valve–mask ventilation Needle thoracocentesis Chest drain placement
Circulation	Control of external haemorrhage	Infusion set up Peripheral venous access ● Extremity veins ● External jugular vein ● Venous cut down Central venous access ● Femoral vein ● External jugular vein Intraosseous access Defibrillation

These practical skills are described in detail in Chapters 21, 22, and 23.

Occasionally it may be appropriate for minor injured people to be treated at the scene, thus avoiding an unnecessary overloading of the hospital system—in such a case it would be sensible to use local general practitioners (but *not* those immediate care doctors with advanced skills) to deliver this treatment.

It is essential that the ambulance, paramedical, nursing, and medical personnel who are sent to the scene of a major incident have current certification at the appropriate level of life support training, as well as having special competence in pre-hospital care. It is totally unacceptable for health service staff attending a major incident response to be either untrained or poorly skilled. Table 17.2 summarises the minimum standards of the various levels that staff should have obtained.

Table 17.2. Minimum training standards

Ambulance officer	MIMMS
Ambulance technician	NHSTD—Extended Ambulance aid
Ambulance paramedic	NHSTD—Paramedic
Hospital doctor	Advanced Trauma Life Support, Advanced Cardiac Life Support, MIMMS
Immediate care doctor	Pre-hospital Emergency Care, MIMMS
Nurse	Advanced Trauma Nursing Course/Trauma Nursing Core Course, Advanced Cardiac Life Support, MIMMS

WHO TREATS?

The problem with the provision of adequate treatment at a major incident is usually not one of lack of staff, but rather one of lack of direction. Everybody from ambulance attendant to senior consultant feels the need to treat rather than to triage or administrate. As discussed earlier in this chapter, treatment is the second step in the hierarchy of medical support. It is absolutely vital that the first step (triage) is used to direct treatment.

Summary
- The first treatment is likely to be basic first aid from unskilled people
- The emergency services are all trained in life saving first aid
- The Ambulance Service has responsibility for treatment on the scene
- Treatment is the second step in medical support
- Attention to airway, breathing, and circulation is most often all that is required at the scene
- All Health Service staff attending major incidents should have current certification at the appropriate level of skill

18

Transport

After reading this chapter you should be able to answer the following questions:

- How are the Casualty Clearing Station and other areas set up to facilitate evacuation and transportation?
- What decisions about transportation need to be made?
- What methods of transportation are available?

INTRODUCTION

Transportation is the third step in the hierarchy of medical support to a major incident. Both triage and treatment decisions will have an effect on transportation. To a large degree the order of evacuation, the destination, and the mode of transportation will be dictated by these earlier decisions.

> **Box 18.1.** The hierarchy of medical support
>
> **T**riage
> **T**reatment
> **T**ransport

As was discussed in Chapter 13, one of the prime tasks of the Health Service command and control structure is to ensure that the movement of patients is as smooth and efficient as possible. To achieve this, close attention needs to be paid to the organisation of transportation both at the scene and beyond. The structure of the treatment and evacuation areas is crucial, as are decisions regarding evacuation methods. Furthermore, the officers responsible for transportation need to have the ability to be flexible about methods of transport and the order of evacuation, if the best use is to be made of limited resources.

ORGANISATION

Two separate aspects need to be considered. The first is the organisation of the chain of transportation for evacuation, while the second is the movement of casualties at the scene.

Chain of transportation

A schematic representation of the ambulance circuit is shown in Figure 18.1.

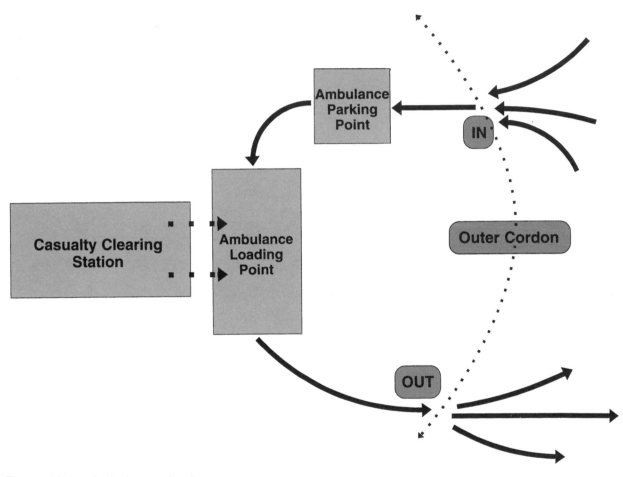

Figure 18.1. Ambulance circuit

Ambulances (and other vehicles if appropriate) will approach the scene from a variety of sources. At the outer cordon they will come under Police control at the incident control point and will be directed to the Ambulance Parking Area. The Ambulance Parking Officer will hold vehicles in this location until notified that they are required by the Ambulance Loading Officer. Once called forward vehicles will proceed to the Ambulance Loading Point (which will usually be adjacent to the Casualty Clearing Station), and will load their assigned casualties. The Ambulance Loading Officer will inform the crew of the casualty's condition, treatment requirements en route, and destination. Once released from the loading point ambulances will proceed around the circuit to a release point at the outer cordon. From here they will proceed to their destination. This system ensures that both the number and nature of vehicles at the loading point are optimised. Incidentally, it also allows the parking area to be used to provide some rest and recuperation for the ambulance crews without interfering with the evacuation process.

132

Casualty flow

To optimise the movement of casualties from the site to receiving hospitals, some patients may bypass the Casualty Clearing Station, whereas others may be held there to ensure that those who reach hospital early are those with the best chance of survival. Two possible schemes are shown in Figures 18.2 and 18.3.

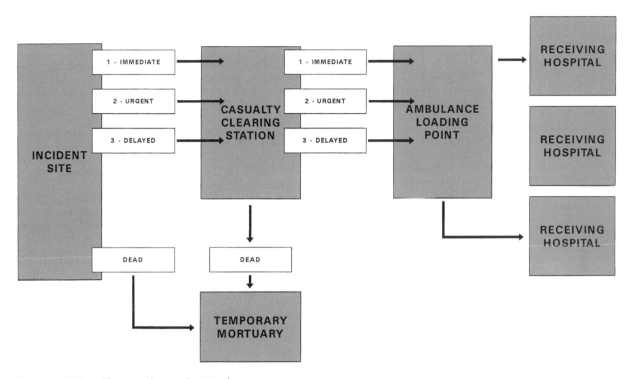

Figure 18.2. Evacuation scheme 1

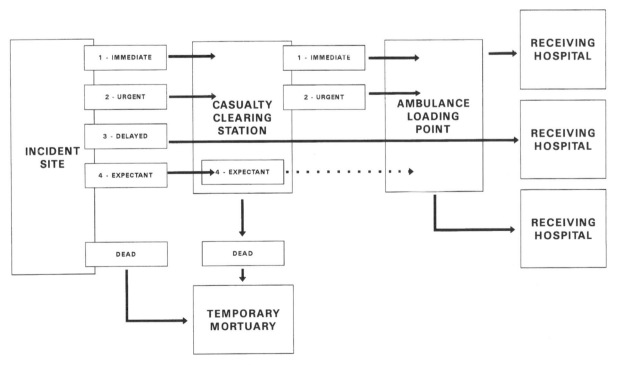

Figure 18.3. Evacuation scheme 2

In the first scheme, the Casualty Clearing Station is the evacuation route for all patients leaving the site. The triage sort occurs in this area and casualties are evacuated with the most serious going first.

In the second scheme, the casualties identified as Priority 3 (delayed) during the triage sieve (that is, those who are walking) are moved directly to the loading area. The patients who are Priority 1 (immediate) and Priority 2 (urgent) (that is, the stretcher cases) are moved to the Casualty Clearing Station and from there to the loading point.

The choice of scheme will greatly affect the transport chain because the numbers of patients arriving at the Ambulance Loading Point, and their priorities, will differ depending on which scheme is used—the scheme shown in Figure 18.3 is recommended because it optimises patient flow for transportation. The first casualties to be available for evacuation will be Priority 3 (delayed) walking wounded. Non-ambulance transport can be used to remove these rapidly to hospital. This phase can occur while the Priority 1 cases are being moved to the clearing station for stabilising treatment, and while ambulances are being mobilised to the scene. By the time these ambulances arrive the initial Priority 1 (immediate) patients are likely to be ready for transportation.

The appropriate use of Priority 4 (expectant) is important at this stage if the best overall outcome is to be achieved.

> **Priority 4 (expectant) patients are considered for transport after Priority 1 patients and before Priority 2 patients**

If Priority 4 (expectant) is used these patients should be transported to hospital after the Priority 1 patients have left the scene.

EVACUATION DECISIONS

There are three key decisions to be made before a particular patient is moved from the scene: the first concerns triage priority, the second treatment and other packaging for evacuation, and the third destination.

Triage priority

Generally the priority for evacuation will be exactly the same as the priority after treatment. The triage sieve and triage sort techniques described in Chapter 16 can be used to determine the priorities in the Casualty Clearing Station. The Secondary Triage Officer and the Ambulance Loading Officer may, however, have to use additional criteria to decide the order of evacuation. The availability of suitable transport and the capacity of vehicles leaving for particular destinations are examples of factors that might be taken into account.

> **Although triage category in the evacuation area is reached using standard triage principles, other criteria have to be taken into account when deciding the exact order in which patients leave the scene**

For example, some casualties may be able to sit, and it would therefore be reasonable to evacuate them from the site using non-emergency ambulances or minibuses. Other patients may be so seriously injured or ill that they need to be transported alone in state of the art emergency vehicles. Still other casualties who have relatively low priorities, but who need to be transported to particular facilities, may leave with a high priority casualty bound for the correct destination.

Treatment and packaging

Various treatments have been discussed in Chapter 17 and are described in detail in Chapters 21, 22, and 23. The correct amount of treatment is that necessary to ensure safe transportation of a casualty to hospital or, if stabilisation is not possible, the amount that will give the casualty the best chance of surviving to reach hospital.

> **Treatment and packaging should be limited to that necessary to allow transport**

The amount of packaging is similarly limited to that necessary for safe transport. A further consideration, which applies particularly for Priority 2 (urgent) casualties, is that rapid transportation to hospital in a major incident does not necessarily ensure rapid assessment and treatment. In such circumstances it may be better for patients to spend more time at the scene. The Medical Incident Officer should be in contact with the various receiving hospitals, and should be able to advise the Casualty Clearing Officer if such delays are necessary.

Destination

It is the responsibility of the Ambulance Incident Officer to decide which hospitals are to be used as receiving hospitals. The Medical Incident Officer will assist by suggesting how many patients of each triage category should be sent to each hospital.

In larger urban areas, where there is a choice of destination, it is better to select patients for specialist facilities at the scene of an incident. The Medical Incident Officer must advise the Ambulance Incident Officer as to which patients are suitable for direct transfer to specialist units.

> **Casualties requiring specialist centres should be transported to them directly from the scene**

Thus a patient who has a severe head injury can be triaged to a neurosurgical centre, and patients with burns can be sent to regional burns units. The rarer the condition or circumstance the more important it becomes to target the patients at the appropriate specialist centre, even though this may initially appear the more difficult course.

METHODS OF TRANSPORTATION

Emergency ambulances

The prime method of transportation from scene to receiving hospital is by emergency ambulance. Such vehicles are specifically designed to enable safe transport of the seriously ill and injured, and have many facilities for the provision of advanced life support en route. In a major incident, when normal Health Service responses are overwhelmed, there may not be enough of these vehicles, and other methods of transportation need to be considered.

135

Other land vehicles

Three key elements must be considered by the Ambulance Incident Officer when transportation needs and possibilities are being assessed (Box 18.2). First, what capacity is needed, and what capacity does each possible vehicle have? Second, what is the availability of each of the possible vehicles? Finally, how suitable are the various possible vehicles for the task in hand? This last decision needs to be based on an assessment of the speed, safety, reliability, and levels of equipment. A wheeled ambulance, for example, will be unsuitable for rough terrain when access roads are limited (unless it is four wheel drive), and tracked vehicles may have to be used or a helicopter considered. It is likely that a number of vehicles such as Police personnel carriers will be available for the transport of the Priority 3 patients. More seriously ill or injured patients who need to be transported on stretchers present more of a problem in this regard. Non-emergency ambulances may be suitable for the Priority 2 (urgent) patients.

Box 18.2. Criteria for selecting transport

Capacity
Availability
Suitability

Helicopters

Helicopters are becoming increasingly available, but the capacity of those that are specifically designed for casualty transport is tiny. Other aircraft, such as those that can be provided by the armed forces, are rarely routinely fitted for stretcher carrying and vary in both capacity and suitability. Helicopters are most suitable when either road communications are disrupted or the terrain is unsuitable for ambulances.

> **Helicopters are most suitable when road transport cannot be used**

In other circumstances the disadvantages often outweigh the advantages. In particular the lack of dedicated helicopter landing sites at hospitals will mean that a number of secondary ambulance journeys from a distant landing site (such as a school playing field) are necessary.

> **The hazards of secondary transfers often outweigh any advantages of a short flight**

These can prove very hazardous indeed and may obviate any advantage that a short smooth helicopter flight may bring.

Other possibilities

In particular circumstances the use of any other means of transport such as boat or train may be considered. For instance, many major airports are extremely well connected to the rail network. If the area is isolated from the main receiving hospitals or if local hospitals are likely to be unable to cope with the numbers of casualties, then it may be advantageous to move some casualties en masse by rail and retriage them on arrival at a station close to other hospitals.

Summary
- Transportation is the third part of the hierarchy of medical support at major incidents
- Effective organisation of both the ambulance circuit and the flow of patients is vital if evacuation is to proceed smoothly
- The order of patient evacuation depends on triage category and other factors
- Emergency ambulances form the mainstay of transport capacity
- Other vehicles may need to be used when the circumstances are appropriate
- Helicopters have a small part to play, but may prove invaluable in particular circumstances

19

Responsibility for the dead

After reading this chapter you should be able to answer the following questions:

- Who pronounces death?
- Who labels the dead?
- When should the dead be moved?
- Where should the dead be moved to?
- How are the dead identified?

PRONOUNCING DEATH

In the United Kingdom only registered medical practitioners can pronounce death. In some Ambulance Services there are guidelines for paramedics to diagnose death in their day to day practice; these guidelines are by no means widespread and have not been extended to the situation of a major incident. Following diagnosis of death by a paramedic, confirmation by a registered medical practitioner is still required.

At the scene of a major incident it would be usual to regard a casualty as dead during primary triage (the triage sieve) if the casualty does not breathe when the airway is opened (see Chapter 16). The doctor pronouncing death should, however, perform a more conventional examination to include the presence of apnoea, asystole (no palpable pulse), and fixed and dilated pupils.

Where possible death should be pronounced in the presence of a policeman who is the representative of HM Coroner.

LABELLING THE DEAD

It is of great importance that the dead are clearly labelled. If this is not done then medical personnel may be repeatedly taken to a body by emergency service staff, who may be unsure of whether resuscitation is possible.

On confirmation of death a triage label is tied to the patient with the white coloured card uppermost. The information that should be recorded is shown in Figure 19.1. A standard police card is now in use and this is illustrated in Figure 19.2.

```
PROBLEM / MAIN DIAGNOSIS




                       DEAD



              Death Pronounced:
        _____
        Time:_____Date_____
        Name of Doctor:_____
        Signature


        _____
        Witnessed by PC:_____
        Number:_____
        Name:_____
```

Figure 19.1. Triage card record of death

The Medical Incident Officer may appoint an individual doctor to the role of Mortuary Officer, and it will be this doctor's duty to pronounce death, label the bodies on scene, and set up a body holding area in conjunction with the Police.

MOVING THE DEAD

A major incident will often be regarded as a scene of crime. The dead will therefore form part of the forensic evidence, and the position they occupy may be important to a later criminal prosecution. For this reason the dead, or parts of bodies, must not be disturbed without the Coroner's permission. There are two exceptions (Box 19.1).

If a body is to be removed its position should be clearly marked. A photograph can demonstrate this, but to be admissible evidence it should be taken by the Scene of Crimes Officer (SOCO).

In some circumstances it may be necessary to dismember a body, perhaps if it is the only way to gain rapid access to a live casualty. This is performed by a process of joint

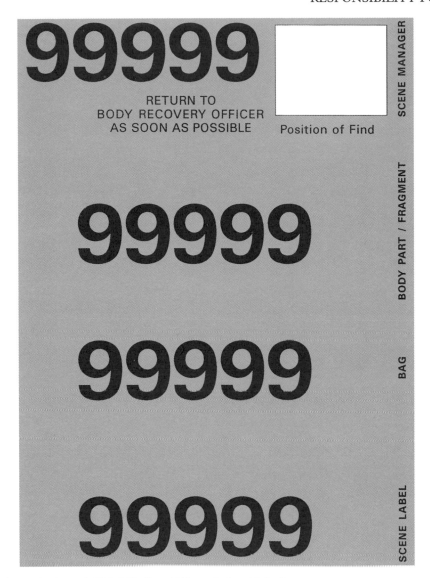

Figure 19.2. Association of Chief Police Officers' dead label

---

Box 19.1. Reasons for moving the dead

To gain access to the living
To prevent destruction by fire or chemicals

---

disarticulation and amputation. Photographs and a description of injuries to the body before it is dismembered will be important.

TEMPORARY MORTUARY

When a body is moved from the point of injury it is taken to a *temporary mortuary* where it can be examined by a forensic pathologist. The facilities to consider when choosing a temporary mortuary are listed in Box 19.2.

The siting of temporary mortuaries should be considered at the planning stage; facilities such as aircraft hangers or ice rinks are ideal. If an incident occurs some distance from a designated area, a *body holding area* will be set up at the scene. This

> **Box 19.2.** The facilities of a temporary mortuary
>
> Capacity for several hundred bodies
> Low ambient temperature
> Adequate sanitation
> Changing and rest areas for staff
> Facility for radiological and other forensic pathology investigations

should be out of sight of the media and the public, and preferably protected from the elements: a school, a village hall, a series of tents, or a number of refrigerated lorries would be options to consider.

All live casualties should be evacuated from the scene before transport is used for the dead.

The dead have the lowest evacuation priority

IDENTIFYING THE DEAD

The Police are responsible for identifying the dead and informing the next of kin. It may be possible to identify the individual from clothing or personal documentation, but this has proved misleading in some incidents when a well wisher has provided the casualty with a coat or other garment. Personal effects such as rings, watches, or wallets should not be removed for safe keeping because this removes vital clues to the individual's identity. When it proves difficult to identify a body by these simple means, techniques such as forensic dentistry will be used.

Information on the identity of people who may have been involved in the incident will be forthcoming from friends and relatives, and this will be collated by the Police Casualty Bureau. Specific questions can be asked of enquirers to help determine the identity of the dead. In the case of most air crashes, information will also be collected by the Emergency Procedures Information Centre (EPIC) based at Heathrow airport. EPIC will work in conjunction with the Police and HM Coroner. When foreign nationals are involved any enquiry from foreign consulates, high commissioners, or embassies will be directed from the Foreign Office to the Casualty Bureau. The Police have a responsibility under the Vienna Convention on Consular Relations to inform these authorities of a death of one of their nationals.

This task of identifying the dead at the scene is undertaken by the Police Identification Commission, under the supervision of the Police Incident Officer.

Summary
- The dead must be labelled
- Only a doctor can pronounce death, and should do so in the presence of a Police officer
- The dead should not be moved unless they prevent access to the living, or the body is in danger of being damaged further
- The Police are responsible for removing bodies from the scene
- The dead will be housed in a *temporary mortuary* for forensic examination, but may have to be held at the scene first in a *body holding area*
- The Police are responsible for identifying the dead and informing the relatives

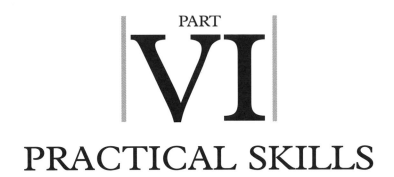

PART
VI
PRACTICAL SKILLS

20

Radio use and voice procedure

After reading this chapter you should understand the techniques used to carry out the following practical procedures and voice procedure (Boxes 20.1 and 20.2):

Box 20.1. Practical procedures

Turn the radio on and transmit a message
Change the radio battery

Box 20.2. Voice procedure

Radio short hand
- Glossary
- Phonetic alphabet
- Numbers and figures

Basic message handling
- Initiate a call
- Replying to a call
- Replying to a group call
- Ending a message
- Offering a message

Advanced message handling
- Corrections
- Repeating a message
- Long message
- Relaying a message

The radio check

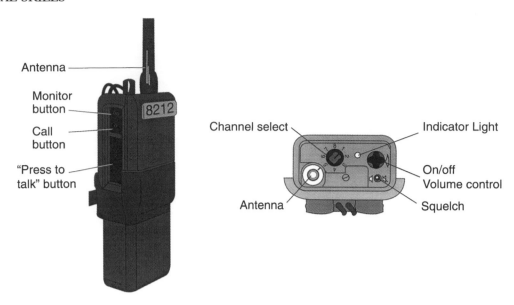

Figure 20.1. The radio working parts

RADIO USE

Turning the radio on and transmitting a message

The reader should refer to Figure 20.1 which shows a hand portable VHF radio.

1 Turn the radio on; many models will produce an audible "beep"
2 Select the channel you require (Box 20.3)

Box 20.3. Channel selection

Channel number	Channel use
1	Emergency reserve (ERC)
2	Local
3	Local
●	●
●	●
69	Emergency services command
Check locally	Local operations

---

3 *Listen* (or *look* at the channel busy light) before transmitting to ensure that the channel is clear
4 Transmit by depressing the "Press to talk" (PTT) button on the side of the radio. Wait one second before starting the message
5 Hold the radio upright and about 4–5 cm from your mouth and speak
6 Release the PTT button to listen to the reply.

Changing the battery

If the messages you receive are crackled or broken, and/or the light flashes during transmission, it is likely that the battery is low. If so, change the battery:

1 Turn the radio off before changing the battery
2 Engage the battery release switch and slide the battery off
3 Slide on the new battery
4 Turn the radio on.

VOICE PROCEDURE

Principles

The fundamentals of a good radio message are:

● Clarity
● Accuracy
● Brevity.

Clarity can be achieved by attention to the following characteristics of the voice:

● Rhythm
● Speed
● Volume
● Pitch.

Remember: RSVP

The *rhythm* should be steady; the *speed* should be slightly slower than normal speech; for adequate *volume* it is not necessary to shout, but do not whisper unless the radio has a specific whisper mode; the best *pitch* is that of a female voice, and men with gruff voices should make a conscious effort to raise their pitch.

To achieve *accuracy* and *brevity* requires discipline and practice. Air time is a valuable commodity. The system of radio voice procedure taught in this book is based on military voice procedure. Examples of alternative systems are given where appropriate.

Radio short hand

Glossary

Brevity can be facilitated by using a number of special words which act as a verbal short hand. These are shown in Box 20.4.

Box 20.4. Special words in radio voice procedure

OVER	The speaker now wishes the receiver to talk
OUT	The conversation is finished
OK	I understand
ROGER	I understand
GO AHEAD	I am ready to receive your message
SEND	I am ready to receive your message
ACKNOWLEDGE	Tell me you have received my message
SAY AGAIN	Repeat what you said
ETA	Estimated time of arrival
ETD	Estimated time of departure
WAIT	I cannot reply within the next five seconds (may be repeated once after five seconds, then WAIT OUT after further five seconds)
WAIT OUT	I cannot reply, I will contact you later
STANDBY	Stay alert, further information to follow

Other words may be in use locally. If so it is essential that their full meaning is known and understood by all users of the net.

The following terminology is *not* acceptable:

- OVER AND OUT   It is either over *or* out
- RODGER DODGER   Slang
- TEN FOUR   Slang.

It is not acceptable to swear on the radio.

The phonetic alphabet

Difficult or important words should be spelt to avoid confusion. Rather than saying "Ay, Bee, See, Dee" a phonetic alphabet is used to give each letter a distinct sound, "Alpha, Bravo, Charlie, Delta." These are shown in Box 20.5.

Box 20.5.   The phonetic alphabet

A	Alpha	N	November
B	Bravo	O	Oscar
C	Charlie	P	Papa
D	Delta	Q	Quebec
E	Echo	R	Romeo
F	Foxtrot	S	Sierra
G	Golf	T	Tango
H	Hotel	U	Uniform
I	India	V	Victor
J	Juliet	W	Whiskey
K	Kilo	X	X-ray
L	Lima	Y	Yankee
M	Mike	Z	Zulu

Key example:

Mike One. Send further supply of ketamine, spell **Kilo–Echo–Tango–Alpha–Mike–India–November–Echo**. Acknowledge over.

Numbers and figures

For accuracy, the pronunciation of numbers is stressed as shown in Box 20.6. Long figures are spoken whole, then repeated digit by digit.

Box 20.6.   Number pronunciation

1	wun	6	six
2	too	7	seven
3	thuree	8	ate
4	fower	9	niner
5	fiyiv	0	zero

> **Key example:**
> Mike One. I require two hundred and fifty, figures too-fiyiv-zero, crepe bandages at the clearing station, over.

Basic message handling

Initiating a call
1 To start a message say "hello" to the station being called
2 Next state who you are
3 Finish the message with "over" (to indicate that the other station can now speak).

> **Key example:**
> Hello Control, this is Mike One, over.

It is also acceptable to initiate a message in the following ways:

Mike One to Control, over.
Control from Mike One, over.

Replying to a call
Prefix each message with the call sign of the station sending the message.

> **Key example:**
> Control. Go ahead, over.
> Mike One. Send resupply of bandages to clearing station, over.

Replying to a group call
Occasionally control or another station will call all the stations on the net. Replies should be in alphanumerical order. Each station is allowed five seconds during which to reply. After this time the next station should reply.

> **Key example:**
> Hello all stations this is control. Acknowledge my last message, over.
> Mike One. Acknowledged, over.
> Mike Two. Acknowledged, over.
> 5 SECOND PAUSE
> Mike Four. Acknowledged, over.
> Control. Mike One, Two and Four acknowledged. Out.

Ending a call
Finish a message with "out." Only one user needs to say "out."

Key example:
Control, OK, over.
Mike One, out.

In some areas Ambulance Control may always have the last word and the following unnecessary transmission will occur after the messages shown above:

Control, base out.

Offering a message
Theoretically, on a constantly monitored radio net it should not be necessary to "offer" a message, that is to say you should be able to move straight into the text of the message. Experience shows, however, that messages *do* need to be offered because the recipient is not always fully alert and may not be in a position to write things down:

1   Initiate the message as shown above
2   Before finishing indicate that a message is to be sent
3   Finish the message with "over" as before.

Key example:
Hello Control this is Mike One. Message, over.

Advanced message handling

Corrections
From time to time you will make errors when sending a message. These errors must be corrected. To correct a message:

1   As soon as an error has been made, say "wrong"
2   Follow this with the correct message
3   If necessary repeat the message for clarity.

Key example:
Mike One. I have now moved to grid thuree-too-wun wun-seven-six.
Wrong. Grid thuree-too-wun *too*-seven six. I say again thuree-too-wun too-seven-six, over.

Repeating
On a military radio net the instruction "say again" is used for a message to be repeated—"repeat" is reserved for artillery to fire again! On a civilian net it is acceptable to say "repeat." To have a message repeated:

1   As soon as the message ends (the sender says "over") reply as shown above
2   Ask for the message to be repeated or said again
3   Finish the message with "over" as before.

> **Key example:**
> Mike One. Say again, over.

If only part of a message need be repeated, then specify which part as shown in Box 20.7.

Box 20.7. Repeating part of a message

Say again all after . . .	Repeat everything after the specified word
Say again all before . . .	Repeat everything before the specified word
Say again all between . . .	Repeat everything between the specified words

---

> **Key example:**
> Mike One. Say again all between PRIORITY and AMBULANCE, over.

Long messages

Occasionally it is necessary to send a long message on the radio. This should be broken down into a series of shorter messages, and the receiver should be asked to acknowledge that they have received each part. Not only does this ensure accuracy, but it gives the opportunity for others on the net to interrupt if they have a more urgent message. Some radios are programmed to stop transmission after a time (for example, 20–30 seconds). Most Ambulance Service systems are not programmed in this way yet. To send a long message:

1 Offer a message as shown above
2 Before finishing indicate that a "long message" is to be sent
3 At frequent intervals (never longer than 30 seconds) ask the receiving station to "acknowledge so far"
4 Repeat any part of the message not received
5 When certain that the message that has been sent already has been correctly received, send the next part of the message
6 Repeat steps 3–5 until all the message has been sent
7 Finish the message.

Relaying a message

If all mobiles are not in contact with control it is sometimes necessary for messages to be passed to one station via another. It is essential that all stages of this process are accurate:

1 The initiator of the message offers a message to an intermediary as shown above
2 Before finishing the initiator indicates that the message is to be passed to another call sign (the final recipient)
3 The message is passed to the intermediary
4 The intermediary acknowledges the message and ends the call with the initiator
5 The intermediary offers a message to the final recipient
6 Before finishing the intermediary indicates that the message is being passed from the initiator
7 The message is passed to the final recipient

151

> **Key example:**
>
> Hello Control this is Mike One, long message, over.
> Control. Go ahead, over.
> Mike One. Require *wun* doctor and nurse team and *too* paramedics to move from the clearing station to the rear coach now, acknowledge so far, over.
> Control. Roger so far, over.
> Mike One. Team to take twenty, figures *too-zero*, bottles of Haemaccel, spell **H**otel–**A**lpha–**E**cho–**M**ike–**A**lpha–**C**harlie–**C**harlie–**E**cho–**L**ima, to give to Forward Incident Officer, acknowledge, over.
> Control. Team to take figures too-zero bottles of Haemaccel, over.
> Mike One, yes. Out.

8　The intermediary ends the call to the final recipient
9　The intermediary calls the initiator and indicates that the message has been passed.

> **Key example:**
>
> Hello Mike One this is Control. Message for Mike Four, over.
> Mike One, send over.
> Control, Message for Mike Four. Send two drug packs to the road, over.
> Mike One, Roger out to you. Hello Mike Four this is Mike One, message from Control over.
> Mike Four, send over.
> Mike One, From Control, send two drug packs to the road over.
> Mike Four, Roger, over.
> Mike One, out to you. Hello Control this is Mike One. Message passed, over.
> Control, Roger out.

The radio check and signal strength

It is important that all stations on any net, and particularly Control, know how good communications are.

This is achieved using the *radio check*: radio checks can be initiated by Control or by other call signs. To perform a radio check:

1　Initiate call to the station or group of stations to be checked
2　Before finishing indicate that a "radio check" is being performed
3　Finish the message with "over"
4　Await the replies
5　Indicate the results of the check to the station or group of stations
6　End the call.

> **Key example:**
>
> Hello Control this is Mike One, radio check, over.
> Control, OK, over.
> Mike One, OK, out.

If communications are not OK then they can be classified as one of the following:

- Difficult—most words are heard but there is interference
- Broken—messages are heard intermittently
- Unworkable—only occasional words are heard—or interference only
- Nothing heard—nothing is heard at all.

152

21

Airway and breathing procedures

After reading this chapter you should understand the techniques used to carry out the following practical procedures:

> Airway opening manoeuvres
> - Chin lift
> - Jaw thrust
>
> Oropharyngeal airway insertion
> - Small child
> - Older child/adult
>
> Nasopharyngeal airway insertion
>
> Orotracheal intubation
> - Infant/small child
> - Older child/adult
>
> Surgical airway
> - Needle cricothyroidotomy
> - Surgical cricothyroidotomy
>
> Ventilation with intubation
> - Mouth to mask ventilation

AIRWAY OPENING MANOEUVRES

Chin lift

Equipment
None (Figure 21.1).

Method
1 Place one hand on the casualty's head to ensure that there is no inadvertent neck movement
2 Place the fingers of the other hand on the bony part of the mandible
3 Lift the bony part of the mandible upwards
4 Reassess the airway by looking for chest movement, listening for the sounds of breathing, and feeling for exhaled air.

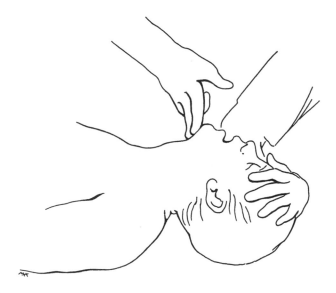

Figure 21.1. Chin lift

Jaw thrust

Equipment
  None (Figure 21.2).

Method
1 Ensure that the casualty's head is maintained in a neutral position
2 Place the little and ring fingers (fourth and fifth digits) of each hand behind the angles of the mandible

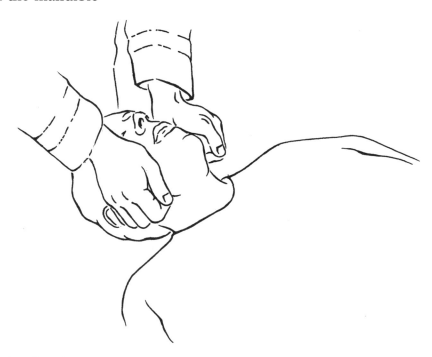

Figure 21.2. Jaw thrust

3 Place the thenar eminences of each hand over the cheek bones
4 Pull the mandible forwards and upwards
5 Reassess the airway by looking for chest movement, listening for the sounds of breathing, and feeling for exhaled air.

OROPHARYNGEAL AIRWAY INSERTION (Figure 21.3)

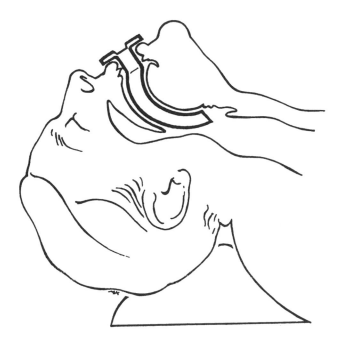

Figure 21.3. Oropharyngeal airway in situ

> **If the gag reflex is present it may be best to avoid the use of an oropharyngeal airway, because such devices may cause choking, laryngospasm, or vomiting**

Small child

1 Select an appropriate size of Guedel airway
2 Open the mouth using the chin lift, taking care not to move the neck if trauma has occurred
3 Use a tongue depressor or a laryngoscope blade to aid insertion of the airway "the right way up"
4 Re-check airway patency
5 If necessary, consider a different size from the original estimate
6 Finally, provide oxygen and consider ventilation by pocket mask or bag and mask.

Older child/adult

1 Select an appropriate size of Guedel airway
2 Open the mouth using the chin lift, taking care not to move the neck if trauma has occurred
3 Insert the airway concave upwards until the tip reaches the soft palate
4 Rotate it through 180° (concave side downwards) and slide it back over the tongue
5 Re-check airway patency
6 If necessary, consider a different size from the original estimate
7 Finally, provide oxygen and consider ventilation by pocket mask or bag and mask.

NASOPHARYNGEAL AIRWAY INSERTION (Figure 21.4)

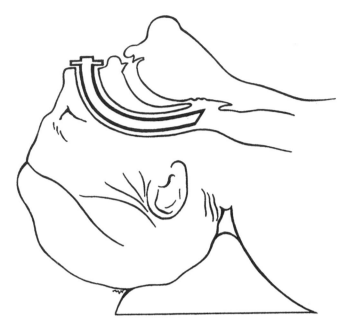

Figure 21.4. Nasopharyngeal airway in situ

Assess for any relative contraindications such as a fracture of the base of the skull.

1 Select an appropriate size (length and diameter)
2 Lubricate the airway with a water soluble lubricant, and insert a large safety pin through the flange
3 Insert the tip into the nostril and direct it posteriorly along the floor of the nose (rather than upwards)
4 Gently pass the airway past the turbinates with a slight rotating motion; as the tip advances into the pharynx, there should be a palpable "give"
5 Continue until the flange and safety pin rest on the nostril
6 If there is difficulty inserting the airway, consider using the other nostril or a smaller size from the original estimate
7 Re-check airway patency
8 Finally, provide oxygen and consider ventilation by pocket mask or bag and mask.

OROTRACHEAL INTUBATION

> **Intubation may be very difficult in the pre-hospital phase of care.**
> **Both the position of the casualty, and the access to him, need to be carefully considered before this procedure is undertaken**

Infant or small child

1 Ensure that adequate ventilation and oxygenation by face mask are in progress.
2 Select an appropriate laryngoscope, and check the brightness of the light.
3 Select an appropriate tube size, but prepare a range of sizes, including the size above and below the best estimate.

> **Endotracheal tube size for children is calculated from their age.**
> **Internal diameter (mm) is 4 plus the age divided by 4**

4   As a result of the relatively large occiput, it may be helpful to place a folded sheet or towel under the baby's back to allow extension of the head.

5   Hold the laryngoscope in the left hand, and insert it into the right hand side of the mouth, displacing the tongue to the left. In the infant, it is sometimes useful to hold the laryngoscope with the left thumb and index and middle fingers, leaving the little finger free to stretch down to press on the larynx to improve the view of the vocal folds. This is particularly useful when performed single handed.

> **Ensure manual immobilisation of the neck by an assistant**
> **if cervical spine injury is possible**

6   In the "flat" baby being intubated by a relatively inexperienced doctor, it is often easiest to place the laryngoscope blade well beyond the epiglottis. The laryngoscope blade is placed down the right hand side of the tongue into the proximal oesophagus. With a careful lifting movement, the tissues are gently tented up to "seek the midline." The blade is then slowly withdrawn until the vocal folds come into view. In some situations, it may be better to stay proximal to the epiglottis to minimise the risk of causing laryngospasm. This decision must be based on clinical judgment.

7   Insert the endotracheal tube into the trachea, concentrating on how far the tip is being placed below the vocal folds. The tip should lie 2–4 cm below the vocal folds depending on age. If the tube has a "vocal fold level" marker, place this at the vocal folds. Be aware that flexion or extension of the neck may cause migration downwards or upwards, respectively.

8   Check the placement of the tube by inspecting the chest for movement and auscultating the chest (including the axillas) and epigastrium.

9   If endotracheal intubation is not achieved in 30 seconds, discontinue the attempt, ventilate and oxygenate by mask, and try again.

Older child/adult

1   Ensure that adequate ventilation and oxygenation by face mask are in progress.

2   Select an appropriate laryngoscope, and check the brightness of the light.

3   Select an appropriate tube size, but prepare a range of sizes, including the size above and below the best estimate.

> **A man requires a size 9 mm tube and a woman a size 8 mm**

4   Hold the laryngoscope in the left hand, and insert it into the right hand side of the mouth, displacing the tongue to the left.

5   Visualise the epiglottis, and place the tip of the laryngoscope in the vallecula.

> **Ensure manual immobilisation of the neck by an assistant if**
> **cervical spine injury is possible**

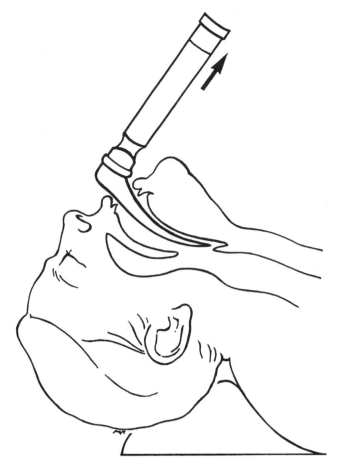

Figure 21.5. Intubation—laryngoscope direction

6 Gently but firmly lift the handle "towards the ceiling on the far side of the room," being careful not to lever on the teeth (Figure 21.5).

7 Insert the endotracheal tube into the trachea, concentrating on how far the tip is being placed below the vocal folds. If the tube has a "vocal fold level" marker, place this at the vocal folds. Be aware that flexion or extension of the neck may cause migration downwards or upwards, respectively.

8 In the adolescent, inflate the cuff to provide an adequate seal. In the pre-pubertal child do not use a cuffed tube.

9 Check the placement of the tube by inspecting the chest for movement and auscultating the chest (including the axillas) and epigastrium.

10 If endotracheal intubation is not achieved in 30 seconds, discontinue the attempt, ventilate and oxygenate by mask, and try again.

Complications of endotracheal intubation include the following:

- Oesophageal intubation (causing severe hypoxia if not immediately recognised)
- Endobronchial intubation, resulting in lung collapse and risk of pneumothorax
- Severe hypoxia from a prolonged attempt to intubate
- Induction of vomiting and risk of aspiration
- Airway injury from the laryngoscope, tube, or stylet (including direct trauma to the vocal folds, as well as chipping or loosening of the teeth)
- Neck strain by over extension, or exacerbation of a cervical spine injury with risk of neurological deterioration

11 A stylet can be used to stiffen the endotracheal tube when intubation proves difficult.

SURGICAL AIRWAY

Cricothyroidotomy is a "technique of failure." It is indicated if a patent airway cannot be achieved by other means. It must be performed promptly and decisively when necessary.

In children under the age of 12 years, needle cricothyroidotomy is preferred to surgical cricothyroidotomy. In the adolescent either technique can be used, but the surgical technique allows better protection of the airway. The relevant anatomy is shown in Figure 21.6.

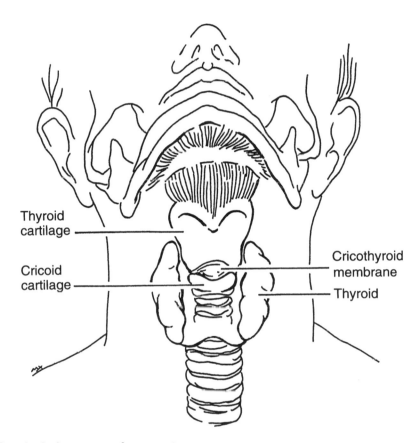

Figure 21.6. Surgical airway—surface anatomy

In a very small baby, or if a foreign body is below the cricoid ring, direct tracheal puncture using the same technique can be used.

Needle cricothyroidotomy

This technique is simple in concept, but far from easy in practice. In an emergency situation the casualty may be struggling, and attempts to breathe or swallow may result in the larynx moving up and down.

1 Attach a cannula over a needle to a 5 ml syringe. Use the biggest cannula appropriate for the size of the patient.
2 Place the patient in a supine position.

3   If there is no risk of cervical spine injury, extend the neck, perhaps with a sandbag under the shoulders.

4   Identify the cricothyroid membrane by palpation between the thyroid and cricoid cartilages.

5   Prepare the neck with antiseptic swabs.

6   Place your left hand on the neck to identify and stabilise the cricothyroid membrane, and to protect the lateral vascular structures from injury from the needle.

7   Insert the needle and cannula through the cricothyroid membrane at a 45° angle caudally, aspirating as the needle is advanced (Figure 21.7).

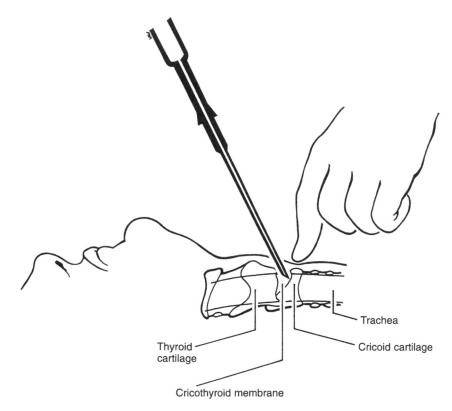

Trachea

Thyroid
cartilage

Cricoid cartilage

Cricothyroid membrane

Figure 21.7.   Needle cricothyroidotomy

8   When air is aspirated, advance the cannula over the needle, being careful not to damage the posterior tracheal wall. Withdraw the needle.

9   Re-check that air can be aspirated from the cannula.

10   Attach the hub of the cannula to an oxygen flowmeter via a Y connector. In a child the initial oxygen flow rate (in litres) should be set at the child's age (in years). In an adult the flow rate should be 12–15 litres/min.

11   Ventilate by occluding the open end of the Y connector with a thumb for 1 second, to direct gas into the lungs. If this does not cause the chest to rise the oxygen flow rate should be increased by increments of 1 litre, and the effect of 1 second's occlusion of the Y connector reassessed.

It is not possible to ventilate a patient via a needle cricothyroidotomy using a self inflating bag. The pressure required to drive gas through the cannula cannot be developed

---

12   Allow passive exhalation (via the upper airway) by taking the thumb off for 4 seconds.

> During trans-tracheal insufflation expiration must occur via the upper airway, even in situations of partial upper airway obstruction. If upper airway obstruction is complete, it is necessary to reduce the gas flow

13 Observe chest movement and auscultate breath sounds to confirm adequate ventilation.
14 Check the neck to exclude swelling from the injection of gas into the tissues rather than the trachea.
15 Secure the equipment to the patient's neck.

Surgical cricothyroidotomy

This should be considered only in adults and older children (12 years or more).

1 Place the patient in a supine position.
2 If there is no risk of neck injury, consider extending the neck to improve access. Otherwise, maintain a neutral alignment.
3 Identify the cricothyroid membrane.
4 Prepare the skin and, if the patient is conscious, infiltrate with local anaesthetic.
5 Place your left hand on the neck to stabilise the cricothyroid membrane, and to protect the lateral vascular structures from injury.
6 Make a small vertical incision in the skin, and press the lateral edges of the incision outwards, to minimise bleeding.
7 Make a transverse incision through the cricothyroid membrane, being careful not to damage the cricoid cartilage.
8 Insert a tracheal spreader, or use the handle of the scalpel by inserting it through the incision and twisting it through 90° to open the airway.
9 Insert an appropriately sized endotracheal or tracheostomy tube. It is advisable to use a slightly smaller size than would have been used for an oral or nasal tube.
10 Ventilate the patient and check that this is effective.
11 Secure the tube to prevent dislodgement.

Complications of cricothyroidotomy include the following:

- Asphyxia
- Aspiration of blood or secretions
- Haemorrhage or haematoma
- Creation of a false passage into the tissues
- Surgical emphysema (subcutaneous or mediastinal)
- Pulmonary barotrauma
- Subglottic oedema or stenosis
- Oesophageal perforation
- Cellulitis

VENTILATION WITHOUT INTUBATION

Mouth to mask ventilation

1 Apply the mask to the face, using a jaw thrust grip, with the thumbs holding the mask (Figures 21.8 and 21.9)
2 Ensure an adequate seal
3 Blow into the mouth port, observing the resulting chest movement
4 Ventilate at 15–30 breaths/min depending on the age of the casualty
5 Attach oxygen to the face mask, if instantly available.

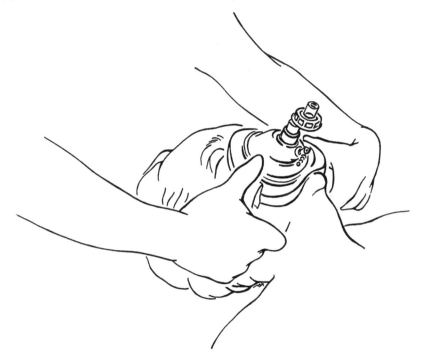

Figure 21.8. Mouth to mask ventilation in an adult

Bag–valve–mask ventilation

1 Apply the mask to the face, using a jaw thrust grip, with a thumb holding the mask (Figure 21.10)
2 Ensure an adequate seal
3 Squeeze the bag observing the resulting chest movement
4 Ventilate at 15–30 breaths/min depending on the age of the casualty.

If a two person technique is used, one rescuer maintains the mask seal with both hands while the second person squeezes the self inflating bag.

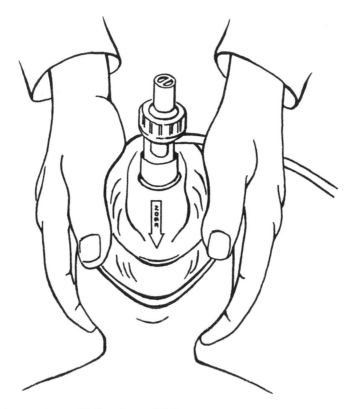

Figure 21.9. Mouth to mask ventilation in a child

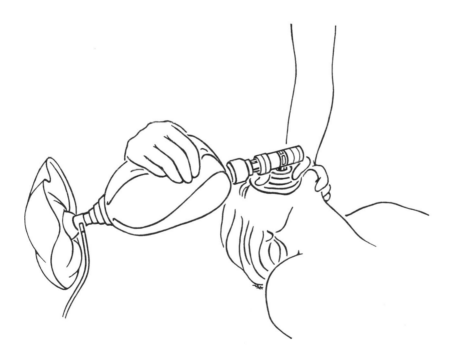

Figure 21.10. Bag and mask ventilation

A reservoir bag should always be used

163

22

Circulatory procedures

After reading this chapter you should understand the techniques used to carry out the following practical procedures:

> *Infusion setup*
>
> *Vascular access*
>   Peripheral venous access
>   upper and lower extremity veins
>   external jugular vein
>   venous cut down
>   Central venous access
>   femoral vein
>   external jugular vein
>   Intraosseous access
>
> *Defibrillation*

INFUSION SETUP

Equipment

1 Infusion fluid
2 Giving set.

> In the pre-hospital setting, particularly during a major incident response where close supervision of both patients and relatively junior rescuers is not possible, it is important to ensure that any interventions are as intrinsically safe as possible. To this end it is recommended that all infusions are airless; this not only reduces the risks of inadvertent air embolus but also allows safe infusion under pressure

Procedure

1 Check the infusion fluid and ensure that it is the correct type and volume, and that it is in date

2   Close the giving set valve and then insert the giving set into the infusion bag
3   Insert the bag and giving set and then open the giving set valve
4   Squeeze the bag, forcing infusion fluid into the upper and lower chambers until they are full
5   Close the giving set valve and then turn the bag and giving set the right way up
6   Slowly open the giving set valve and allow the infusion fluid to flow down the tubing
7   Close the valve once the fluid reaches the patient connector.

> **Once filled in this way the bag can be placed under a patient
> and the fluid infused using the patient's weight to increase flow**

VASCULAR ACCESS

Access to the circulation is a crucial step in delivering Advanced Life Support. Even if conditions are not ideal an effort should be made to ensure that access is obtained with routine cleanliness, and that any infusion that is attached is both safely applied and accurately recorded.

> **Many routes are possible; the one chosen will refect both
> clinical need and the skills of the operator**

Peripheral venous access

Upper and lower extremity veins
   Veins on the dorsum of the hand, the elbow, the dorsum of the feet, and the saphenous vein at the ankle can be used for percutaneous cannulation.
   Standard percutaneous techniques should be employed.

External jugular vein

   Equipment
1   Skin cleaning swabs
2   Appropriate cannula
3   Tape.

   Procedure
1   Place patient in a 15–30° head down position (or with padding under the shoulders so that the head hangs lower than the shoulders)
2   Turn the head away from the site of puncture; restrain the patient as necessary in this position
3   Clean the skin over the appropriate side of the neck
4   Identify the external jugular vein which can be seen passing over the sternocleidomastoid muscle at the junction of its middle and lower thirds
5   Have an assistant place a finger at the lower end of the visible part of the vein just above the clavicle; this stabilises and compresses it so that it remains distended
6   Puncture the skin and enter the vein
7   When free flow of blood is obtained ensure that no air bubbles are present in the tubing and then attach a giving set
8   Tape the cannula securely in position.

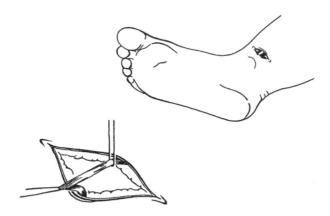

Figure 22.1. Cut down technique

Venous cut down

> If speed is essential it may be more appropriate to use the intraosseous
> route for immediate access in children under 12 (see below),
> and to cut down later for continued fluid and drug therapy

Equipment
1 Skin cleaning swabs
2 Lignocaine 1% for local anaesthetic with 2 ml syringe and 25 gauge needle
3 Scalpel
4 Curved haemostats
5 Suture and ligature material
6 Cannula.

Procedure (Figure 22.1)
1 Immobilise the appropriate limb
2 Clean the skin
3 Identify the surface landmarks for the relevant vein—shown in Table 22.1
4 If the patient is responsive to pain, infiltrate the skin with 1% lignocaine
5 Make an incision perpendicular to the course of the vein through the skin
6 Using the curved haemostat tips, bluntly dissect the subcutaneous tissue
7 Identify the vein and free 1–2 cm in length
8 Pass a proximal and a distal ligature

Table 22.1. Surface anatomy of the brachial and long saphenous veins

	Brachial	Saphenous
Infant	One finger breadth lateral to the medial epicondyle of the humerus	Half a finger breadth superior and anterior to the medial malleolus
Small children	Two finger breadths lateral to the medial epicondyle of the humerus	One finger breadth superior and anterior to the medial malleolus
Older children/adults	Three finger breadths lateral to the medial epicondyle of the humerus	Two finger breadths superior and anterior to the medial malleolus

9   Tie off the distal end of the vein, keeping the ends of the tie long
10 Make a small hole in the upper part of the exposed vein with a scalpel blade or fine pointed scissors
11 While holding the distal tie to stabilise the vein, insert the cannula
12 Secure this in place with the upper ligature; do not tie this too tightly and cause occlusion
13 Attach a syringe filled with 0·9% saline to the cannula and ensure that fluid flows freely up the vein; if free flow does not occur then either the tip of the cannula is against a venous valve (in which case withdrawing it will improve flow) or the cannula may be wrongly placed in the adventitia surrounding the vein
14 Once fluid flows freely, tie the distal ligature around the cannula to help immobilise it
15 Close the incision site with interrupted sutures
16 Fix the cannula or catheter to the skin and cover with a sterile dressing.

Central venous access

Central access can be obtained through the femoral, internal jugular, external jugular, and subclavian veins. In pre-hospital care the femoral vein is often used as it is relatively easy to cannulate and away from the chest during cardiopulmonary resuscitation. It is possible to obtain relatively safe central access via the external jugular vein.

> **Central venous access via the deep neck veins is difficult and may be dangerous in emergency situations even in hospital— it is not recommended during pre-hospital care**

Femoral vein

Equipment
1   Skin cleaning swabs
2   Lignocaine 1% for local anaesthetic with 2 ml syringe and 23 gauge needle
3   Syringe and 0·9% saline
4   Seldinger cannulation set:
    —syringe
    —needle
    —Seldinger guidewire
    —cannula
5   Suture material
6   Prepared infusion set
7   Tape.

Procedure
1   Place the patient supine with the groin exposed and leg slightly flexed and abducted at the hip; restrain the patient's leg and body as necessary
2   Clean the skin around the appropriate side
3   Identify the puncture site; the femoral vein is found by palpating the femoral artery—the vein lies immediately medial to the artery
4   If the patient is responsive to pain, infiltrate the area with 1% lignocaine
5   Attach the needle to the syringe
6   Keeping one finger on the artery to mark its position, introduce the needle at a 45° angle pointing towards the patient's head directly over the femoral vein; keep the

syringe in line with the patient's leg and advance the needle, pulling back on the plunger of the syringe all the time

7   As soon as blood flows back into the syringe, take the syringe off the needle; occlude the end of the needle immediately to prevent blood loss

8   If the vein is not found withdraw the needle to the skin, locate the artery again, and advance as in (6)

9   Insert the Seldinger wire into the needle and the vein

10 Withdraw the needle along the wire, ensuring that the wire is not dislodged from the vein

11 Place the cannula over the wire and advance it through the skin, into the vein

12 Suture the cannula in place

13 Withdraw the wire, occluding the end of the cannula immediately to prevent blood loss

14 Attach the infusion set

15 Tape the infusion set tubing in place.

External jugular vein

By using the Seldinger technique it is possible to obtain central venous access via the external jugular vein as described below. The anatomy is such that passage into the central veins can sometimes be more difficult compared with other approaches.

Equipment
1   Skin cleaning swabs
2   Lignocaine 1% for local anaesthetic with 2 ml syringe and 23 gauge needle
3   Syringe and 0·9% saline
4   Seldinger cannulation set:
    —syringe
    —needle
    —Seldinger guidewire (J wire)
    —cannula
5   Suture material
6   Prepared infusion set
7   Tape.

Procedure
1   Place patient in a 15–30° head down position (or with padding under the shoulders so that the head hangs lower than the shoulders)
2   Turn the head away from the site of puncture; restrain the patient as necessary in this position
3   Clean the skin over the appropriate side of the neck
4   Identify the external jugular vein, which can be seen passing over the sternocleidomastoid muscle at the junction of its middle and lower thirds
5   Have an assistant place a finger at the lower end of the visible part of the vein just above the clavicle; this stabilises the vein and compresses it so that it remains distended
6   Attach the needle to the syringe and puncture the vein
7   As soon as free flow of blood is obtained, take off the syringe and occlude the end of the needle
8   Insert a J wire into the needle and the vein
9   Advance the J wire; there may be some resistance as the wire reaches the valve at the proximal end of the vein, so gently advance and withdraw the wire until it passes this obstacle
10 Continue to advance the wire gently

169

11 Withdraw the needle along the wire, ensuring that the wire is not dislodged from the vein
12 Place the cannula over the wire and advance it through the skin, into the vein
13 Suture the cannula in place
14 Withdraw the wire, occluding the end of the cannula immediately to prevent air embolism
15 Attach the infusion set
16 Tape the infusion set tubing in place.

Intraosseous transfusion

The technique of intraosseous infusion is not new. It was used in the 1930s as a quick method of gaining vascular access (the only alternatives were to use a reusable, resharpened metal needle or to perform a venous cut down). As it is important to achieve vascular access quickly in many life threatening situations, intraosseous infusion is again being recommended. Specially designed needles make this quick and easy. It is indicated if other attempts at venous access fail, or if they will take longer than five minutes to carry out. It is contraindicated if there are fractures proximal to the proposed site of access.

Equipment
1 Alcohol swabs
2 18 gauge needle with trochar (at least 1·5 cm in length)
3 5 ml syringe
4 50 ml syringe
5 Infusion fluid.

Procedure
1 Identify the infusion site; fractured bones should be avoided, as should limbs with fractures proximal to possible sites. The landmarks for the upper tibial and lower femoral sites are shown Table 22.2, and the approach to the tibial site is illustrated in Figure 22.2
2 Clean the skin over the chosen site
3 Insert the needle at 90° to the skin
4 Continue to advance the needle until a give is felt as the cortex is penetrated
5 Attach the 5 ml syringe and aspirate to confirm correct positioning
6 Attach the filled 50 ml syringe and push in the infusion fluid in boluses.

Table 22.2. Surface anatomy for intraosseous infusions

Tibial	Femoral
Anterior surface, 2–3 cm below the tibial tuberosity	Anterolateral surface, 3 cm above the lateral condyle

DEFIBRILLATION

To achieve the optimum outcome defibrillation must be performed quickly and efficiently.

Many defibrillators are available. Providers of Advanced Life Support should make sure that they are familiar with those they may have to use.

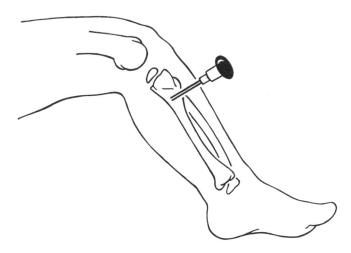

Figure 22.2. Tibial technique for intraosseous infusion

> **Requirements for optimum defibrillation:**
> **Correct paddle position**
> **Correct paddle placement**
> **Good paddle contact**
> **Correct energy selection**

Correct paddle selection

Most defibrillators are supplied with adult paddles attached (13 cm diameter or equivalent area); 4·5 cm diameter paddles are suitable for use in infants, and 8 cm diameter are used for small children.

Correct paddle placement

The usual placement is anterolateral. One paddle is put over the apex in the midaxillary line, and the other is placed just to the right of the sternum, immediately below the clavicle (Figure 22.3).

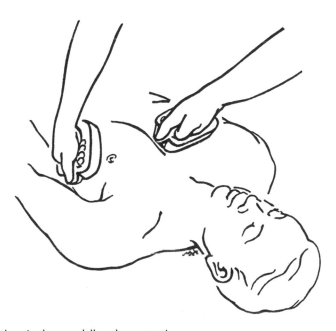

Figure 22.3. Standard anterior paddle placement

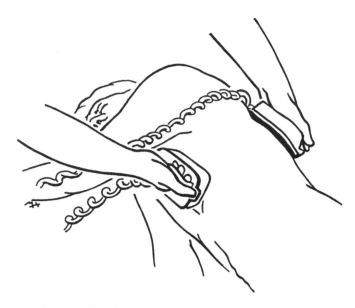

Figure 22.4. Anteroposterior paddle placement

If the anteroposterior placement is used, one paddle is placed just to the left side of the lower part of the sternum, and the other just below the tip of the left scapula (Figure 22.4).

Good paddle contact

Gel pads or electrode gel should always be used (if electrode gel is used, care should be taken not to join the two areas of application). Firm pressure should be applied to the paddles.

Correct energy selection

The levels recommended by the European Resuscitation Council should be used.

Safety

The user must ensure that other rescuers are not in physical contact with the patient (or the stretcher or trolley) at the moment the shock is delivered.

> **Defibrillators deliver enough current to cause cardiac arrest. Safety is paramount**

Procedure
1 Apply gel pads or electrode gel
2 Select the correct paddles
3 Select the energy required
4 Press the charge button

Basic life support should be interrupted for the shortest possible time

5 Wait until the defibrillator is charged
6 Place the electrodes onto the pads of gel, and apply firm pressure
7 Shout "Stand back!"
8 Check that all other rescuers are clear
9 Deliver the shock.

CHAPTER
23
Trauma procedures

After reading this chapter you should understand the techniques used to carry out the following practical procedures:

> *Chest decompression*
>   Needle thoracocentesis
>   Chest drain placement
>
> *Femoral nerve block*
>
> *Spinal care*
>   Cervical spine immobilisation
>   application of a cervical collar
>   application of sandbags and tape
>
>   Logrolling
>   application of a long spine board
>   Rapid extrication

CHEST DECOMPRESSION

Needle thoracocentesis

This procedure can be life saving and can be performed quickly with minimum equipment.

Needle thoracocentesis must be followed by chest drain placement

Minimum equipment
1 Alcohol swabs
2 Large over the needle intravenous cannula (16 gauge and larger)
3 20 ml syringe.

Procedure
1 Identify the second intercostal space in the midclavicular line on the side of the pneumothorax (the *opposite* side to the direction of tracheal deviation)
2 Swab the chest wall with surgical prep solution or an alcohol swab
3 Attach the syringe to the cannula
4 Insert the cannula into the chest wall, just above the rib below, aspirating all the time
5 If air is aspirated remove the needle, leaving the plastic cannula in place
6 Tape the cannula in place and proceed to chest drain insertion as soon as possible.

> **If needle thoracocentesis is attempted, and the patient does not have a tension pneumothorax, the chance of causing a pneumothorax is 10–20%. Patients who have had this procedure must have a chest radiograph and will require chest drainage if ventilated**

Chest drain placement

Chest drain placement should be performed using the open technique described here. This minimises lung damage. In general, the largest size drain that will pass between the ribs should be used. In the pre-hospital setting it is essential that the drainage apparatus itself is able to withstand some trauma, and that it is easily transportable.

> **For pre-hospital care the drainage apparatus must be robust and easily transportable**

For these reasons chest drainage bags rather than bottles are recommended. Heimlich valves are robust enough, but often stick because of blood and serosanguineous fluids—they are not recommended.

Minimum equipment
1 Skin prep solution
2 (Local anaesthetic)
3 Scalpel
4 Scissors
5 Large clamps ×2
6 Chest drain
7 Chest drainage bag
8 Suture.

Procedure
1 Decide on the insertion site (usually the fifth intercostal space in the midaxillary line) on the side with the pneumothorax
2 Swab the chest wall with surgical prep solution or an alcohol swab
3 Use local anaesthetic if necessary
4 Make a 2–3 cm skin incision along the line of the intercostal space, just above the rib below
5 Bluntly dissect through the subcutaneous tissues just over the top of the rib below, and puncture the parietal pleura with the tip of the clamp
6 Put a gloved finger into the incision and clear the path into the pleura
7 Advance the chest drain tube into the pleural space

176

8   Ensure that the tube is in the pleural space by listening for air movement and looking for fogging of the tube during expiration
9   Connect the chest drain to the drainage bag
10 Suture the drain in place and secure with tape.

FEMORAL NERVE BLOCK

The femoral nerve supplies the femur with sensation and consequently a femoral nerve block is useful in cases of femoral fracture. The technique may also be of benefit when analgesic drugs (such as morphine) would interfere with the management or assessment of other injuries.

A long acting local anaesthetic agent should be used so that splinting and other management can be undertaken with minimal distress to the casualty. If a rapid effect is required (for example, for extrication) then a shorter acting anaesthetic agent such as lignocaine should be used.

Femoral nerve block can be carried out even if opiates are contraindicated

Equipment
1   Antiseptic swabs to clean
2   Lignocaine 1%
3   10 ml syringe
4   Needle
5   Bupivicaine 0·5%.

Procedure
1   Move the fractured limb gently so that the femur lies in abduction and the ipsilateral groin is exposed
2   Swab the groin clean with antiseptic solution
3   Identify the femoral artery and keep one finger on it; the femoral nerve lies immediately lateral to the artery
4   Infiltrate the skin just lateral to the artery with lignocaine (Table 23.1); aspirate the syringe frequently to ensure that the needle is not in a vessel
5   Inject the chosen anaesthetic agent around the nerve, taking care not to puncture the artery
6   Wait until anaesthesia occurs (bupivicaine may take up to 20 minutes to have its full effect).

Table 23.1.   Volume of local anaesthetic for femoral nerve block

	Age (years)		
	>12	5–12	<5
Bupivicaine 0·5% volume (long action) (ml)	10	5	1 ml/year
Lignocaine 1% (rapid onset) (ml)	20	10	2 ml/year

SPINAL CARE

Cervical spine immobilisation

All casualties with serious trauma must be treated as though they have a cervical spine injury. It is only when adequate investigations have been carried out and any necessary neurosurgical or orthopaedic consultation completed that the decision to remove cervical spine protection can be taken.

> **There will never be adequate resources at the scene to allow cervical injury to be excluded**

In line cervical stabilisation, as shown in Figure 23.1, should be applied until a hard collar has been applied and sandbags and tape are in position as described below. Both techniques are described and it is necessary to use both to achieve adequate cervical spine control.

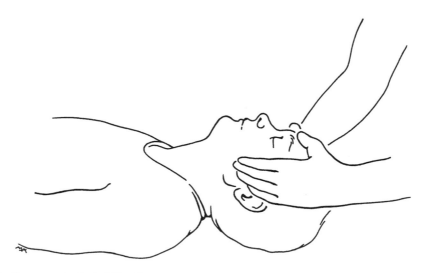

Figure 23.1. In line cervical stabilisation

Application of a cervical collar

Minimum equipment
1 Measuring device
2 Range of hard collars.

> **The key to successful, effective collar application lies in selecting the correct size**

Method
1 Ensure that in line cervical stabilisation is maintained throughout by a second person
2 Using the manufacturer's method, select a correctly sized collar

178

3   Fully unfold and assemble the collar
4   Taking care not to cause movement, pass the flat part of the collar behind the neck
5   Fold the shaped part of the collar round and place it under the casualty's chin
6   Fold the flat part of the collar with its integral joining device (usually Velcro tape) around until it meets the shaped part
7   Reassess the correct fit of the collar
8   If the fit is wrong, slip the flat part of the collar out from behind the neck, taking care not to cause movement; select the correct size and recommence the procedure
9   If the fit is correct secure the joining device
10   Ensure that in line cervical stabilisation is maintained until sandbags and tape are in position.

Application of sandbags and tape

Equipment (Figure 23.2)
1   Two sandbags
2   Strong narrow tape.

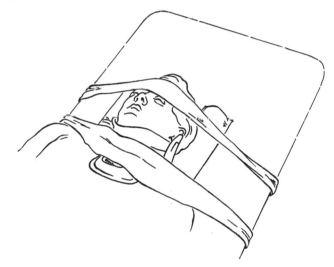

Figure 23.2. Sandbags, hard collar, and tape

Method
1   Ensure that in line cervical stabilisation is maintained by a second person throughout
2   Place a sandbag either side of the head
3   Apply tape across the forehead and attach it securely to the long spinal board
4   Apply tape across the chin piece of the hard collar and attach it securely to the long spinal board.

> *Exceptions to the rule:*
> Both the frightened uncooperative casualty and the casualty who is hypoxic and combative may paradoxically have increased cervical spine movement if sandbags and tape are applied. This is because these casualties will fight to escape from any restraint. In such cases a hard collar alone should be applied, and no attempt made to immobilise the head

Logrolling

To minimise the chances of exacerbating unrecognised spinal cord injury, non-essential movements of the spine must be avoided. If manoeuvres that might cause spinal movement are essential (for example, moving a casualty on to a long spine board or during examination of the back at the secondary survey) then logrolling should be performed. The aim of logrolling is to maintain the orientation of the spine during turning of the casualty.

> **The basic requirements for successful logrolling are an adequate number of rescuers and good control**

Method
1 Gather together enough staff to roll the casualty: in larger children and adults four people will be required; three will be required in smaller children and infants
2 Place the staff around the patient as shown in Table 23.2
3 Ensure that each member of staff knows what he or she is going to do (Table 23.3)
4 Carry out essential manoeuvres as quickly as possible.

Table 23.2. Staff positions during logrolling

	Size of casualty	
Staff member	Smaller child and infant	Larger child and adult
1	Head	Head
2	Chest	Chest
3	Legs and pelvis	Pelvis
4		Legs

Table 23.3. Staff tasks during logrolling

Staff member position	Task
Head	Hold either side of the head (as for in line cervical stabilisation), and maintain the orientation of the head with the body in all planes during turning *Control the logroll by telling other staff when to roll and when to lay the casualty back on to the trolley*
Chest	Reach over the casualty and carefully place both hands over the chest. When told to roll the casualty, support the weight of the chest and maintain stability. Watch the movement of the head at all times and roll the chest at the same rate
Pelvis and legs	*This only applies to smaller children and infants. If it is not possible to control the pelvis and legs at the same time get additional help immediately* Place one hand either side of the pelvis over the iliac crests. Cradle the child's legs between the forearms. When told to roll the child grip the pelvis and legs and move them together. Watch the movement of the head and chest at all times, and roll the pelvis and legs at the same rate
Pelvis	Place one hand over the pelvis and the other under the patient's leg. Watch the movement of the head and chest at all times and roll the pelvis at the same rate
Legs	Support the weight of the legs either by placing both hands under them, or by holding them on each side. When told to roll the casualty watch the movement of the chest and pelvis and roll the legs at the same rate

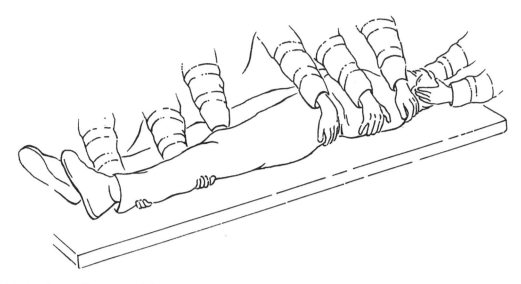

Figure 23.3. Logrolling an adult

Application of a long spine board (Figure 23.4)

Minimum equipment
1 Long spinal board
2 Securing straps
3 Head blocks or other head immobilisation device.

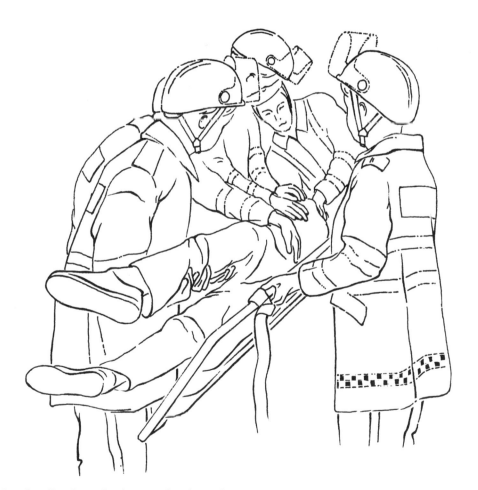

Figure 23.4. Application of a long spine board

Method

1 Gently move the head into neutral alignment
2 Logroll the casualty (see above)
3 Place the long spinal board next to the casualty; the board can be placed flat on the ground, at an angle, or flat against the patient's back, the last minimising the spinal movement, but requiring more rescuers
4 Logroll the casualty back onto the board (if the board was against the casualty's back or at an angle to it, the patient and the board are lowered together)
5 Taking care not to cause spinal movement, position the casualty in the centre of the board
6 Immobilise the upper body on to the board
7 Immobilise the lower body on to the board
8 Pad under and around the head as necessary, place head blocks (or an alternative such as rolled up blankets) either side of the head, and immobilise by strapping over the forehead and across the cervical collar
9 Immobilise the legs on the board
10 Place the casualty's arms by the side and secure them.

Rapid extrication

The technique described is that for a sitting casualty.

> **Rapid extrication is indicated if the scene is unsafe, if the casualty's condition is such that life saving interventions are necessary (and cannot be performed *in situ*), or if the patient is blocking access to a casualty with life threatening injuries**

Minimum equipment
1 Cervical collar
2 Long spine board.

Method
1 Gather together enough staff to perform the procedure; in adults and children a minimum of three people will be necessary
2 Place the staff as shown in Table 23.4.

Table 23.4. Staff positions during rapid extrication

Staff member	Position
1	Head
2	Left
3	Right

This may mean that one or more rescuers are inside a vehicle, building, or other structure.

3 The first rescuer brings the head to a neutral position
4 A second rescuer (the one on the side to which the casualty is to be moved) supports the patient's chest

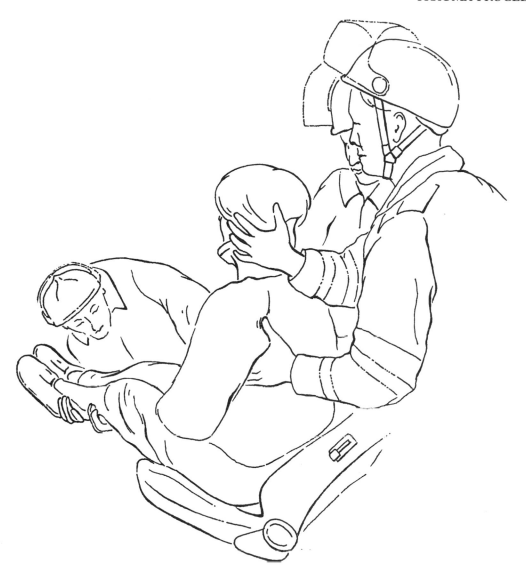

Figure 23.5. Rotating the patient

5   The casualty is moved to the sitting position
6   After a rapid assessment the cervical collar is applied
7   A third rescuer (the one on the side away from which the casualty is to be moved) ensures that there are no obstacles preventing movement of the patient's lower body and legs

> **Spinal control will be lost if the complete rotation is carried out in one movement**

8   The casualty is rotated bit by bit until facing away from the desired direction of movement; in line stabilisation of the cervical spine is maintained throughout (Figure 23.5).
9   A long spinal board is inserted under the upright patient

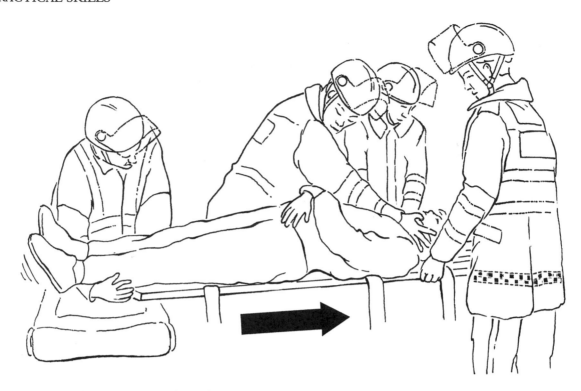

Figure 23.6. On to the spine board

10 The patient's upper body is lowered on to the board
11 While in line stabilisation is maintained the patient is slid along the board until centred on it (Figure 23.6).

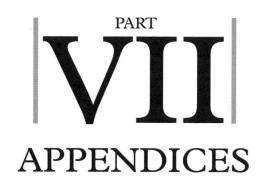

PART

VII

APPENDICES

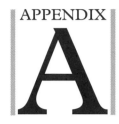

APPENDIX

A

Special incidents

This appendix will consider the special circumstances surrounding a major incident in each of the following situations:

- Chemical spillage
- Radioactive contamination
- Multiple burns casualties
- Mass gatherings

CHEMICAL SPILLAGE

Safety

In the event of an incident involving a chemical spillage always think of safety first—your own, that of those approaching the scene, and the safety of any casualties (the *1–2–3 of safety*). You must not attempt to reach and treat those inside the contaminated area until it has been declared safe by the Fire Service. In the event of a chemical incident:

CALL OUT   the Fire Service
GET OUT   of the immediate vicinity
STAY OUT   of the contaminated area until it has been made safe.

**Think of safety to begin,
If injured you're no use to him**

Identification of the hazard

You can obtain information on the nature of the chemical from the information displayed on the plate at the rear of the tanker, or on the outside of a loose drum. This information should be passed to Fire Service Control. There are two systems in current use on British roads—the United Kingdom Hazard Identification System (UKHIS, often referred to as "HAZCHEM"), and the European "Kemmler" system.

The UKHIS plate

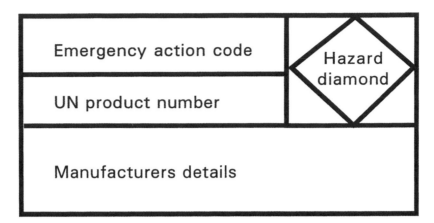

Figure A.1. The UKHIS plate

This is illustrated in Figure A.1. There are four elements:

1 The emergency action code
2 The United Nation's product number
3 The hazard diamond
4 Manufacturer's details.

The first figure of the emergency action code tells the Fire Service how to fight the fire, whether with jets, fog, foam, or dry agent. The middle letter indicates what protective clothing must be worn when dealing with the hazard, and whether it must be contained or can safely be washed into the storm drains. If the letter "E" is present at the end of the code, this means "consider evacuation." The medical team should *stay clear until it is declared safe to approach.*

> **When "E" is on the hazard plate,**
> **Always think "Evacuate!"**

The United Nation's product number is used to identify the exact nature of the chemical, and provide first aid advice. The information can be obtained from central fire control or in some authorities via facsimile ("CHEMDATA") on the pumping appliances.

The hazard diamond gives a colour-coded warning as to the nature of the hazard, together with a written warning, such as "corrosive" or "flammable liquid."

The manufacturer's telephone number is listed for supplementary advice to the Fire Service in the event of a spillage.

The Kemmler plate

This is illustrated in Figure A.2. There are two elements:

1 A numerical hazard identification
2 The United Nation's product number.

The numerical hazard lists the primary hazard first, then lesser hazards. If a number is repeated, this means that the hazard is intensified. For example:

3	Flammable liquid
33	Highly flammable liquid
333	Spontaneously flammable liquid
333X	Spontaneously flammable liquid which reacts violently with water

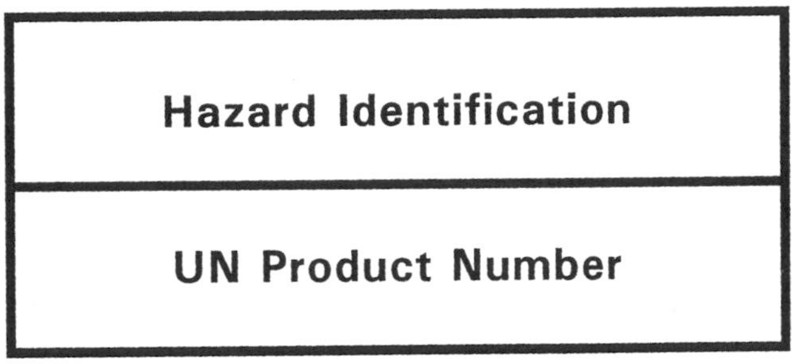

Hazard Identification

UN Product Number

Figure A.2. The Kemmler plate

The United Nation's product number is the same as that on the UKHIS plate.

**A Kemmler number that is double,
Means a hazard twice the trouble**

TREM card

The Transport Emergency card, or TREM card, is carried in the driver's cab of a chemical tanker. It lists the exact nature of the chemical being transported, together with brief actions in the event of a spillage, including first aid and specific antidotes.

**Get at the TREM card if you can,
It has first aid for the fireman**

Poisons centres

The poisons information centres will provide a valuable advisory service for the hospital response to large numbers of chemical casualties, and can also provide a service to identify chemicals (at the scene this is the responsibility of the Fire Service) and to determine from where antidote can be obtained (and arrange its delivery).

Medical responsibilities at the scene

The MIO must ensure the following:

- Adequate clothing and protection of himself and his medical teams
- Decontamination of the casualties
- Appropriate treatment and transfer to hospital of casualties.

Doctors and nurses are not immune from the effects of chemicals. Medical staff *must not* enter a contaminated area to treat casualties unless they are wearing the necessary protective clothing. Casualties should be decontaminated and passed into a "clean"

189

area before treatment; this area should not be exposed to recontamination from the principal hazard (for example, indoors/under tentage to protect from vapour cloud). If there is an overriding clinical need for treatment, the casualty may be attended to before decontamination *but only if the medical staff have appropriate personal protection equipment.* These medical staff should not re-enter the clean area until they too have been decontaminated. Decontamination at the scene is usually restricted to removing clothing (seal in a plastic bag) and washing with cold water. The Fire Service decontamination shower is a high pressure shower in which the firefighter stands (with his breathing apparatus) on his way out of the contaminated area; it is rarely suitable for casualties.

The Casualty Clearing Station should be sited up hill and up wind of a chemical hazard, when this is possible.

If a chemical incident threat is identified in an area, it would seem prudent for the medical staff who will be sent to the scene to train specifically for dealing with contaminated casualties.

Medical responsibilities at the hospital

Decontamination facilities must also be provided at the hospital. Staff must be protected from cross contamination by wearing appropriate clothing. The following key points should be considered:

- A patient with physical and chemical injury will have a poorer prognosis than with the physical injury alone
- Associated physical injuries are common
- Respiratory symptoms following inhalation of noxious substances are often delayed for up to 24–48 hours
- Patient should not be discharged back into the contaminated environment.

At the hospital a Chemical Assessment Team (CAT) can be formed whose responsibilities are outlined in Box A.1.

Box A.1. Responsibilities of the Chemical Assessment Team (CAT)

Identify the toxic chemical contaminants
Assess the level of contamination
Assess the risk of contamination to other patients and staff
Assess the adequacy of decontamination (patients and staff)
Assess the contamination of the "dirty" area, and advise on its return to normal use

---

RADIOACTIVE CONTAMINATION

It is realistic to anticipate radioactive contamination in a civilian setting in the following circumstances:

- Spillage of medical isotopes in transit
- Accident at a nuclear power installation (contained)
- Accident at a nuclear power installation (uncontained; home or abroad)
- Accident involving nuclear waste or fissile material in transit
- Accident involving nuclear warheads in transit or at a military establishment.

It is not within the scope of this text to predict the probability of each of these events. The priorities of the medical service at the scene of radioactive contamination are, as ever, safety of yourself first, then to protect others from becoming contaminated, then to deal with the contaminated casualties—the *1–2–3 of safety.*

If there is a radioactive source do not approach the scene. Wait for the Fire Service to declare the area safe.

An individual who has simply been exposed to a radiation source without contamination poses no threat to his rescuers and should be treated along standard resuscitation guidelines. He will not "emit" any radiation himself (unless he has *ingested* a considerable quantity of radioactive substance). It is useful to remember that the primary emission from uranium or plutonium is α rays, which are blocked by intact skin.

A casualty who has surface contamination can usually be dealt with by removal of clothes and washing the areas exposed to the contaminant dust. Any residual dust after this procedure is unlikely to be a significant threat to the rescuers. If there is no immediate access to monitoring equipment it should be assumed that the casualty is contaminated and any staff dealing with these casualties *must* wear appropriate protective clothing.

A radiation incident is always a "major incident" in the eyes of the public, no matter how small the contamination or how negligible the risk, and intense media interest should be anticipated. The primary source of advice on the management of such an incident will be the medical physics department in the nearest hospital which is listed as providing assistance under the National Arrangements for Incidents Involving Radiation (NAIR). Such a hospital should provide the necessary monitoring equipment to assess the level of contamination and the adequacy of decontamination.

In the event of a large number of people being exposed to a radioactive source the military can be approached to provide specialist advice and assistance with casualty treatment, as could the occupational health department of a civil nuclear installation. Gastrointestinal symptoms are a common and early consequence of those who require hospital observation. The prognosis for conventional injuries is made worse by concomitant radiation exposure, and the triage category for treatment should take this into account.

At hospital a Radiation Assessment Team (RAT) can be formed with the responsibilities listed in Box A.2.

Box A.2. Responsibilities of the Radiation Assessment Team (RAT)

Confirm the nature of the radiation source, and its component risks
Assess the level of radioactive contamination
Assess the risk of contamination to other patients and staff
Assess the adequacy of decontamination (patients and staff)
Assess the contamination of the "dirty" area, and advise on its return to normal use

---

MULTIPLE BURNS CASUALTIES

Incidents involving a large number of casualties with burns injuries pose a particular problem with the disposal of the injured from the scene, because the expertise to deal with burns injuries is concentrated in a relatively small number of centres nationally. This is compounded by the need to recognise those who may require intensive care facilities within the next 12–24 hours, because this is also a limited resource within each hospital.

It is well known that doctors inexperienced in the assessment of burns will often make an inaccurate assessment of the size of the burn (more often over estimating the size), and additionally they may be unfamiliar with the warning signs of respiratory involvement or with a fluid resuscitation formula. It may seem logical to send a burns expert to the scene to assist with triage, but this is unlikely to be practical as casualties will usually not be trapped (those trapped in a fire will die of smoke inhalation) and therefore will be moved rapidly from the scene before such an expert could be mobilised.

Alternatively, all casualties could be sent to the regional burns unit for assessment. This would mean, however, that a considerable number of minor burns (which could be dealt with in a district hospital) *and* a number of unsalvageable patients would divert the valuable resources of the burns surgeons away from those who can benefit the most. As the fundamental principle of major incident casualty management is to "do the most for the most," this does not appear to be a satisfactory solution.

The final, and probably the best, option is to pulse casualties to a number of hospitals so that no single unit is overwhelmed. Each hospital can be visited by a Burns Assessment Team (BAT), consisting of a burn specialist (registrar grade or above) and a burns nurse, who will identify those who require specialist treatment, either in terms of burns surgery or elective ventilation, and advise on the early management of other burns casualties.

Direct triage from the scene to a regional burns unit should, therefore, weed out those with a minor burn or those who will certainly die. These groups should be sent to the district general hospital(s). The Burns Assessment Team will provide a secondary triage tier for those who were incorrectly categorised at the scene. It is generally accepted that when the sum of the percentage burn and the casualty's age (the burns index) exceeds 100, then the chance of survival approaches zero (although the premorbid state should also be taken into consideration); with a respiratory component to the burn the prognosis is worse. Table A.1 gives a suggested tool for the triage officer at the scene for those casualties aged 15 years and over.

Table A.1. Triage for mass burn casualties ($\geqslant$15 years only)

Age + percentage burn	Send to
<35	District general hospital
35–100	Regional burns unit
>100	District general hospital

Those with respiratory burns should also be identified at the scene and sent to a hospital with an available intensive care bed. All children would best be managed in a paediatric burns unit, but in the event of large numbers of children those with minor burns ($\leq$10–15% surface area burn) could be managed in a district hospital with a paediatric surgical facility. The BAT can also advise on those adults or children with small burns to "specialist" areas (for example, hands, perineum, eyes, over large joints) which require the skills of a burns surgeon.

MASS GATHERINGS

In the last few years there has been an increased emphasis on mass gathering medical support, as a result of a number of major incidents and their subsequent well publicised reports. For example, recommendations made by Lord Justice Taylor following the Hillsborough football stadium tragedy in 1989 have led to the appointment of a safety officer (full or part time) at every football ground in the country.

Planning

Mass gatherings present special difficulties for major incident planning. A stadium may have a population of 45 000 for 2–3 hours every weekend, but is empty for the remainder of the week. The result, in many instances, is a failure to recognise the potential for catastrophe. This shows itself as a failure to provide a detailed Major Incident Plan, an absence of regular training, and a paucity of funding.

An effective Major Incident Plan will be based on detailed prior knowledge of the site. This should involve all aspects of both internal and external geography, potential trouble spots, and the surrounding road and rail systems. A knowledge of the local hospitals and the probable availability of general and specialised beds is also important. Access and egress routes for ambulances, including the Ambulance Parking Point, should be preplanned to facilitate the smooth flow of casualties.

An effective medical plan can only be formulated after close liaison with the Police, Fire, and Ambulance Services. At those events where the St John Ambulance Service or the Red Cross are involved in routine medical support, then they should also be represented in the planning phase so that their role in a major incident is clearly defined.

Training

The Health Service personnel present at a mass gathering event will be from a variety of backgrounds. A general training in safety, access, communications, and triage is essential. Additional training should be directed towards specific roles.

Ancillary staff such as football match stewards may be given training beyond simple first aid (such as triage), and may then have an important role in the medical plan.

Summary
- Incidents may be special because of the substances involved, the type of injuries caused, or the location
- The principles of medical management still apply
- Assessment is particularly important
- The principles of medical support still apply

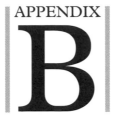

Psychological aspects of disasters

This appendix will consider the psychological effects of disasters as they affect both the rescuers and the rescued. Three stages will be discussed:

> - Immediate
> - Early
> - Late

INTRODUCTION

Psychological problems are common in the injured, in uninjured survivors, and in those involved with the rescue operation following a major incident. Many more people than are physically injured can be expected to have a psychological injury. The psychological aspects will be considered here in terms of immediate, early, and late problems.

> **Psychological problems are common.**
> **They occur in the injured, uninjured survivors, and the rescuers**

IMMEDIATE

Initially both the injured and the uninjured survivors may be understandably anxious and upset about their injuries, or about having narrowly missed being killed. These people may also be upset about friends and relatives who have been killed or injured, or who are missing.

It is less common for the rescuers to be overcome by the situation because, hopefully, they will be part of a coordinated and ordered response. Each Incident Officer should, however, be alert to the signs of stress and fatigue in his workers and be prepared to withdraw affected individuals from the scene.

EARLY

Survivors may feel guilty at having lived through the experience when a friend or relative has died, or blame themselves for their death or injury: *"If I hadn't wanted to go to London that day..."* Equally, those injured may feel anger and resentment towards a perceived guilty party. Such emotions should be anticipated and help offered. Follow up can be particularly difficult. For example, an uninjured survivor of a transport disaster may be discharged from hospital, return some distance home, and suffer such feelings in isolation.

Health Service staff who are used to dealing with suffering on an individual basis may be overwhelmed by the magnitude of the human disaster. No one is immune, but junior staff can be particularly vulnerable.

Efforts must be made to offer psychological debriefing to all those involved through the general practitioner, hospital departmental head, community psychiatric nurse, or psychiatric social worker. The emergency department consultant may wish to hold a short debriefing for his staff after the "stand down" has been announced, but more importantly there should be a formal debriefing session within 48 hours, after people have had a chance to consider the events. Open discussion, irrespective of position, should be encouraged.

> **Anticipate problems and pre-empt them with adequate, early debriefing**

LATE

Those exposed to a major incident may suffer the symptoms of *post-traumatic stress disorder* (PTSD). These symptoms may persist for years if untreated. This is more common when there has been a deliberate attempt to kill an individual (such as a terrorist bomb). Warning signs include unpleasant flashbacks or nightmares, poor work performance, anxiety, depression, or fear of associated events (such as travelling on a train after a rail incident). Formal psychiatric help may be needed.

> **Summary**
> - Psychological effects may be immediate, early, or late
> - Planned intervention will minimise adverse reactions in both patients and staff

196

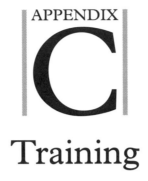

APPENDIX

C

Training

This appendix will consider the following questions:

> ● Why is training necessary?
> ● How is training carried out?

THE NEED TO TRAIN

This book has shown that the environment and the skills required for optimal performance at major incidents are quite different to those with which most Health Service professionals are familiar. To be able to perform adequately at both the scene of a major incident and at receiving hospitals therefore requires training.

HOW TO TRAIN

Training can be considered in terms of education and exercise. The MIMMS course provides the Mobile Medical Team members and the Incident Officers with knowledge that they can apply to the medical management and support of any major incident.

The actual treatment of patients in the pre-hospital environment is taught on a number of courses. A Pre-Hospital Emergency Care Certificate is awarded by the Royal College of Surgeons of Edinburgh and the Pre-Hospital Trauma Life Support Course is run by the Royal College of Surgeons of London. The Diploma in Immediate Medical Care from the Royal College of Surgeons of Edinburgh tests the candidates' knowledge of major incident management with a rigorous practical examination, including a triage exercise and a table top major incident. Advanced life support skills for patient treatment are taught on Advanced Trauma Life Support, Advanced Cardiac Life Support, and Advanced Paediatric Life Support courses and these treatment principles are, on the whole, transferable to a major incident environment.

Major incident education is more, however, than simply the treatment skills for large numbers of traumatised patients. It must include instruction on command and control, radio communications, interservice liaison, and how the scene of an incident is structured. This is provided by MIMMS.

Higher education is available in the form of a Civil Emergency Planning Certificate (University of Bradford) or a Master of Science degree in Civil Emergency Planning (University of Hertfordshire). The Society of Apothecaries have recently introduced a Diploma in Military and Civil Catastrophes.

Exercises

Major incident exercises are an important part of the preparation for an incident. The types of exercise are listed in Box C.1.

Box C.1. Types of training exercise

Paper triage exercise
Dynamic triage exercise
Communications exercise
Table top exercise
Departmental exercise with casualties
Practical exercise without casualties
Interservice exercise with casualties

Paper triage exercise

Trainees are asked to triage a number of casualties having been given enough clinical information about each. This is best done by identifying whether the casualties are immediate, urgent, delayed, expectant, or dead rather than by assigning a numerical order of intervention. Paper exercises can incorporate as much background information and incidental training as the instructors deem necessary. For instance, the layout and command structure can be re-emphasised.

Dynamic triage exercise

A similar scenario is used to the paper exercise, but trainees must respond as a group to each casualty, as the casualty is encountered. Thirty seconds are given for the trainees to read the information on a single casualty before the group responds simultaneously by lifting up a triage label of the appropriate colour. Differences of opinion can then be discussed. This method encourages rapid decision making in the initial triage sieve at a major incident.

Communications exercise

These exercises will specifically test the trainees' ability to use a radio, and aim to give them confidence and authority when using this communication tool. Call in methods can be exercised in this way.

Table top exercise

A table top exercise will allow the trainees to discuss the overall management of the scene and to observe how the medical service integrates with the other emergency services. This is ideally done with representatives from each of the emergency services.

Departmental exercise with casualties

A number of mock casualties are made up and fed into the system. The exercises test the ability of particular departments to handle casualties. They can be carried out without disrupting other departments, and without detriment to the service for those with conventional illnesses and injuries. The exercise may be extended into as many parts of the hospital as required, but will not involve any pre-hospital response.

Practical exercise without casualties (PEWC)

A PEWC is designed to test command and control skills in the pre-hospital environment. Trainees are taken to the area in which an imaginary incident has taken place and posed a number of problems (for example, Where should the Casualty Clearing Station be sited? Where would you park the ambulances?). The problems are solved both individually and after group discussion.

Interservice exercise with casualties

These large exercises may occur on an annual basis and provide an opportunity to practise the whole Major Incident Plan within hospitals and outside. There is a statutory requirement for certain installations (for example, airports and chemical installations) to practise their plan regularly, and advantage should be taken of this to run a concomitant hospital exercise. Small scale exercises take place regularly (every 1–2 months), usually organised by individual emergency services. The medical services may observe or send a small pre-hospital response to practice sessions if this is deemed appropriate.

Summary
- Training is essential if the response is to be optimal
- Individual and group training should be undertaken
- Many training methods are available; those chosen should reflect both training aims and the needs of the participants

Index